YOGA
WEEK BY WEEK

By the same author with Elisabeth Haich

Yoga and Health
Over 1,500,000 copies sold. Translated into eighteen languages
Yoga and Destiny
Raja Yoga

By Selvarajan Yesudian
A Yoga Miscellany
Self-Reliance Through Yoga

By Elisabeth Haich
Initiation
Sexual Energy and Yoga
The Wisdom of the Tarot

All published by George Allen & Unwin Ltd

YOGA
WEEK BY WEEK
Exercises and meditations for all the year round

SELVARAJAN YESUDIAN

Translated by D. Q. Stephenson

With a Foreword by Elisabeth Haich

London   GEORGE ALLEN & UNWIN LTD

Ruskin House   Museum Street

This translation © George Allen & Unwin Ltd 1975

Originally published in German under the title *Hatha Yoga Ubungsbuch*
© Drei Eichen Verlag Hermann Kissener 1971

ISBN 0 04 149024 x hardback
ISBN 0 04 149025 8 paperback

Printed in Great Britain
in 11 pt Baskerville type by
Cox & Wyman Ltd
London, Fakenham and Reading

*I dedicate this book to all
sincere practitioners of Yoga*

Foreword

In *Yoga and Health*, the first book on which we collaborated, Selvarajan Yesudian presented the simple classical Hatha Yoga exercises which anyone here in the West—irrespective of age or health—can practise safely and successfully. Many pupils have been doing these exercises for a number of years, and it therefore became necessary to suggest additional exercises to make the body still more vital and conscious of itself. With affectionate care Selvarajan Yesudian has selected fresh exercises which will be of benefit to his pupils and enable them to achieve a still greater measure of success and obtain even better results. He has embellished the many different exercises with tasteful drawings and poems so as to endue them with still greater vitality of form. The whole work breathes Yesudian's loving spirit with its delicate and truly oriental quality. No photograph could be a better likeness of Yesudian than this book of exercises. A picture would show merely his earthly likeness, his earthly features; but this book is an image of his inner nature woven from love and benevolence. This book will afford everyone using it a true and inward joy, just as I myself rejoiced to see the pleasure and zeal with which Selvarajan Yesudian put together this book of exercises for the Yoga School which he holds dear above all else.

I present this work to the practitioners of Yoga with all my affection.

Elisabeth Haich

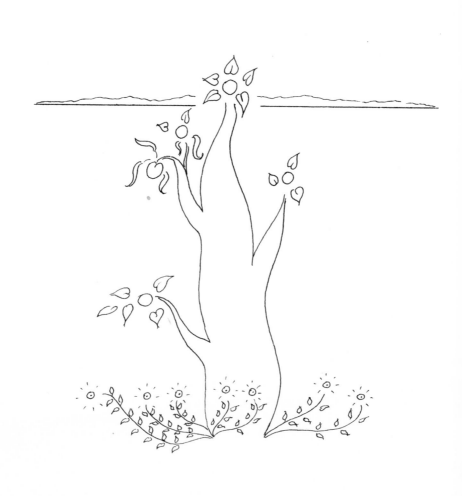

Preface

Since Elisabeth Haich and I published our book *Yoga and Health* in several languages, the interest in Yoga has grown to such an extent that the time has come for a new book containing additional Hatha Yoga exercises. The breathing exercises and asanas (body postures) have proved to be of the greatest prophylactic and therapeutic value. Today many doctors and psychiatrists recommend their patients to practise correct breathing and Yoga exercises as a vital part of their treatment. This book contains more practice than theory—it is intended to be a practical pointer to radiant health: the mirror and realisation of a controlled way of thinking. Without either the one or the other there can be no happiness.

To have a thorough knowledge of Yoga the reader should be familiar with some chapters of *Yoga and Health* such as 'What is Hatha Yoga', 'The Constructive Power of Consciousness', 'Complete Breathing', 'Every Disease has Mental Causes', etc.

Purity of mind and body is of great importance for those who would practise Yoga. This is why I have compiled a page of sublime thoughts selected from the great thinkers for each set of exercises. Whether these be read with full awareness or not, they penetrate deep into our subconscious mind, take root there, and gradually become part of our being. They inculcate wisdom in what we think and do, and so, without our knowledge, they purify our soul.

It gave me special pleasure to pen the little drawings. Through them I have been able to give subtle expression to a great deal I could not have put into words. Words can be found for trains of thought, but often a state of being can be expressed better in a small sketch than in a description.

Although parts of this book were originally written in English, it was first published in German under the title of *Hatha Yoga Ubungsbuch* (Drei Eichen Verlag, München). The author is deeply indebted to Mr D. Q. Stephenson for revising the original English texts and translating the rest of the book from the German.

I would ask my reader to accept this modest work in the same spirit of love as that in which I hand it to my dear Yoga friends.

Selvarajan Yesudian

Contents

1 Some Thoughts to Ponder

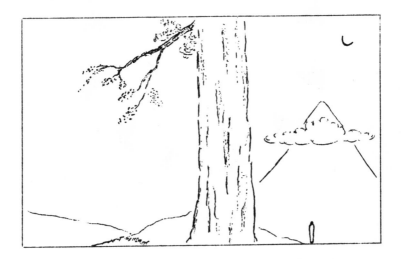

Who is man's great teacher? None other than man himself. Is it not he who reads the enigmatic signs at the cross-
roads of life, advancing his steps from birth to birth? Are
not his senses sufficient to enable him to speak his earthly
tongue? Does he not come a traveller equipped for the
long journey of life? What mystery does the casket of his
brain conceal? And is his heart not hidden away so that
none can know what treasure it contains? Like a seed
yielding its possession of a mighty tree, so too does man
yield the divinity he conceals. We may clothe his naked
form for a while, we may strengthen his limbs with food,
we may shed some earthly light on his human path, but in
the end it is he who grows by giant steps, it is he who speaks
the immortal tongues, and it is he who vanishes when his
play is played.

S.Y.

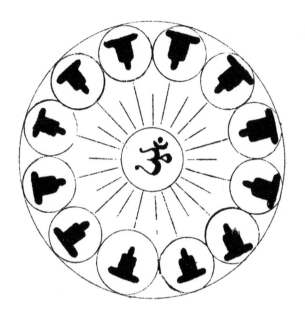

A human being attains perfection by mastering his senses.
Is there anything that is impossible for him who has
mastered his passions?

Ramakrishna

It is easy for a good man to do good but difficult for a
wicked man. It is easy for a wicked man to do evil but
difficult for a good man.

Buddha

Just as the greatest wind cannot move a solid rock, so
neither calumny nor praise can move a wise man.

Buddha

The higher we fly, the smaller we seem to those living on
the earth.

Nietzsche

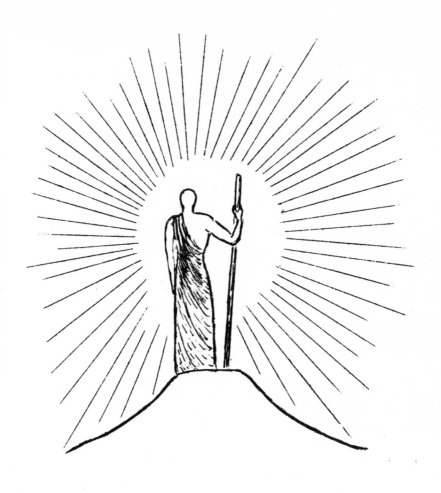

The more circumstances are against you, the more your inner strength becomes manifest.

Vivekananda

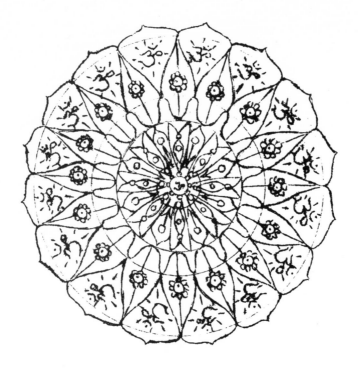

Can condemning this world amend matters? It brings nothing but confusion. Show the path leading out of darkness, and man will readily follow. Faith is the foundation-stone of life. Remove it and life itself crumbles.

Just as a mighty ocean remains unruffled by a little breeze, so the strength of the man of spirit is unaffected by human weakness.

S.Y.

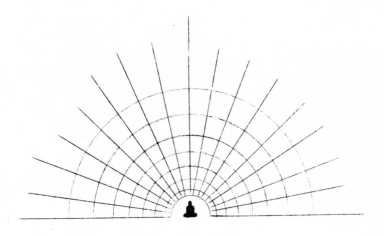

Eternity calls!
Arise and sleep no more!
Life's a dream
Which began yesterday
And will end tomorrow.
Arise!
Awake!
And sleep no more!

S.Y.

Consciousness is a state of the SELF. As consciousness grows, there will unfold in us all the latent qualities which Buddha, Jesus of Nazareth, Ramakrishna, Vivekananda and other giants of the spirit made manifest.

Patience is the keyword in Yoga, patience attended by diligence and perseverance. If various prophets have succeeded in manifesting their divine nature, it is in the power of every man and woman to do the same.

Hatha Yoga is not a science of the body. Hatha Yoga takes the body merely as a starting point. We develop physical strength which is automatically converted into intensity of feeling, power of understanding, and finally into energy of spirit. First, then, we pass beyond the bodily plane, and extend our consciousness to the plane of understanding, and finally we unfold it in its unbounded, unlimited, free form, as spiritual consciousness. Our joy at our growing consciousness we experience as a state of happiness.

S.Y.

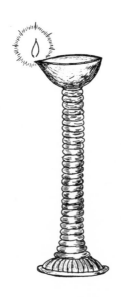

Thousands of years ago there lived a sage named Yajnavalkya. He had two wives called Maitreyi and Kalyani who were very dear to his heart. Kalyani was worldly-minded and cared chiefly about the ordinary pleasures of life. She looked after the household, and her interests did not extend beyond the limits of everyday existence. Maitreyi, however, thought a great deal about things which concerned the inner life and loved to learn more of truth.

One day the sage called his two wives to his side and said: 'The span of earthly life is short. What a man must know of life I have already learnt, but what he must know of truth I have still to learn. Grant me leave to retire from worldly life, so that the rest of my years are not spent in vain. As a dream fades, so life passes. Let me depart with your blessings. The house I leave to you both, the lands are yours to enjoy, the cattle are yours, and so is all my silver and gold.'

Kalyani consented to this arrangement, but Maitreyi was unhappy at the prospect. With tears in her eyes, she addressed her husband thus: 'This world is indeed like a dream. For even if one has wealth, can one obtain freedom? For all one's possessions, can one be sure of happiness? In the midst of many pleasures, can one attain knowledge? And from the endless cycle of life and death, can one expect liberation? Dispel my doubts, my lord, and help me to see the truth. If immortality is the goal of the human spirit, what have I to do with the short-lived pleasures of life?'

'O my Maitreyi, you were always dear to my heart, but now you are more precious than ever,' said Yajnavalkya. 'Come, sit by my side and I will teach you the truth. Truth is first heard of, then seen, and at last realised. Listen, and you too shall know the truth.

'Do you know why we cherish the things we love in this world, my Maitreyi? The spirit that pervades all creation pervades the things we love, hence we cherish the spirit in the things we love.

'Never for the sake of the husband does the wife love the husband, but for the sake of the Self in him she loves him, for she loves the Self.

'Never for the sake of the wife does the husband love the wife but for the sake of the Self in her he loves, for he loves the Self.

'Never for the sake of the child do the parents love the child, but they love the Self in the child.

'Never for the sake of wealth do we love wealth, but for the sake of the Self in wealth, for we love the Self. In all things created the Self is inborn, hence we love the Self in all creation.

'As a mirror reflects the sun, so do this earth and the universe reflect the Self, and thus we love the Self in all created things. Likewise we love the scriptures, for the Self is contained in them, hence we love the Self in the scriptures.

'O my Maitreyi, see the Self in all things. The tree is beautiful because the spirit is beautiful in the tree. The mountains are beautiful because the spirit is beautiful in the mountains. The spirit must first be heard of, then seen, then meditated upon. Know the Self, and you know all else. Know that the spirit is the origin of all creation. But the spirit can be seen only in its manifestation, for the spirit itself is eternal and knows no beginning and no end.

'Just as the sound of the drum cannot be grasped with the hands, but when the drum is held the sound can be controlled, so too the meaning of this world can be grasped only when the Self is known.

'As smoke spreads in all directions from a lighted fire, so the knowledge of the scriptures issues from the Being of all beings.

'As the sun pours its bright rays in every direction, so the light of truth issues from that Being of all beings.

'As the skin knows all the feelings of touch, as the nose recognises all odours, the eyes perceive all forms, the ears distinguish all sounds, so the Self is the repository of the myriad created beings in this world, to which all life returns in the end as the rain returns to the ocean.

'As light when it falls banishes all darkness, so the spirit knows no imperfection.'

After imparting this knowledge to Maitreyi, he arose, blessed his wives and departed.

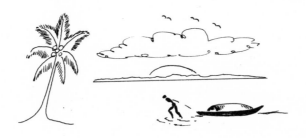

2 The Fifty-two Guiding Thoughts for the Fifty-two Tables of Exercises

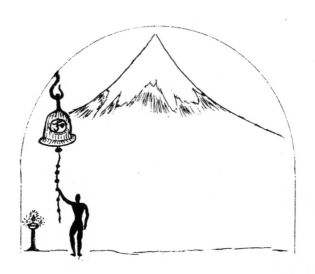

Let bold and fearless thoughts take shape in your brain, and let each breath you breathe, each word you speak, and all your deeds be imbued by these thoughts. That is the way to convert weakness into strength, serfdom into freedom, and what is deadly into what gives life.

S.Y.

One should pay no heed to the words of men. No one could ever achieve greatness in life if he allowed their praise or censure to affect him.

Vivekananda

I do not want a teacher who influences me. What I want is a teacher who teaches me not to let myself be influenced.

S.Y.

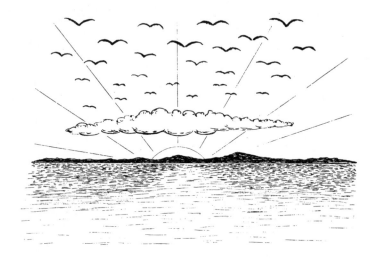

Only the youngest novices need time specially set aside
for their meditations. The advanced student gradually
feels an ever-waxing sense of happiness whether he works
or not. While his hands are busy in the community, he
keeps his head cool in solitude.

Ramana Maharshi

The Self

The Self is unique. Motionless, it is quicker than thought. The senses cannot overtake it, for it always has a start over them. Standing still, it overtakes everything that moves. Without the Self there can be no life.

The fool thinks that the Self moves, but it does not move. To the fool it seems remote, but it is close. It is within everything and yet outside everything.

He who sees all living beings in his Self and his Self in all living beings can no longer hate.

Illumination means: to find one's own Self in the whole universe. He who sees unity everywhere has vanquished delusion and care.

The Self is omnipresent, radiant, without a body, without bones, without flesh, perfect, pure and untouched by evil. The seer, the thinker, the One, the highest over all the world whose being is self-sustained and who has created the world for all eternity.

O Sun, the face of truth is obscured by thy golden disc. Withdraw that I, the seeker after truth, might see the glory of truth.

Preserver thou, Seer, Ruler of Heaven and Earth—O radiant Sun, thou source of life to all creatures—cover up thy light, and gather in thy rays! Let thy lovely form see me through thy grace. The indwelling essence in thee is I.

The secret of immortality is plumbed only by he who is pure in heart when, in the profoundest meditation, he recognises this: The Self in me and Brahman (the Absolute) outside are one. To be one with God, that is immortality!

The Upanishads

If you carry round with you thoughts of ill will, hate or anger, their destructive force will tell upon your own body and your own soul. The harm they will do you is indescribable. The yogis say that thought is the greatest power in the body, greater than the word, for it is a transcendental power that infuses the whole world. Good thoughts, however unimportant they may seem, will not fail to achieve their effect. Have courage and know that you create your own fate. Think sound thoughts, utter sublime thoughts, such as you would like to see realised at the level of action. With perseverance you will soon master your thoughts, which will then help instead of hinder you. Instead of sowing irresponsible thoughts which poison your own life and that of those you meet, master your thoughts and be aware of the power you possess. Then you will come to see the reality of Vivekananda's words: If matter is mighty, then thought is almighty.

S.Y.

'Reproach no man with imperfections', taught our master; 'do you not see that he is taking the greatest trouble to make progress—be it ever so little?'

S.Y.

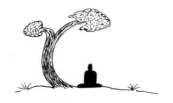

I want sappers and miners in my army of religion! So boys, set yourselves to the task of training your muscles! For ascetics, mortification is all right. For workers, well-developed bodies, muscles of iron and nerves of steel!

Vivekananda

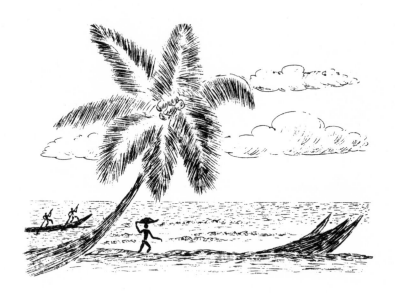

It is the greatest manifestation of power to be calm. It is easy to be active. Let the reins go, and the horses will run away with you. Anyone can do that, but he who can stop the plunging horses is the strong man. Which requires the greater strength, letting go, or restraining? The calm man is not the man who is dull. The calm man is the one who has control over the mind waves. Activity is the manifestation of inferior strength, calmness of the superior.

Vivekananda

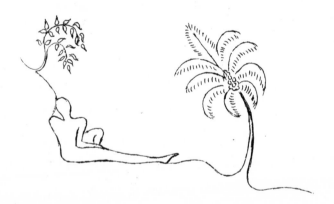

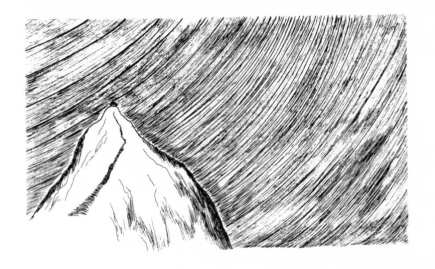

Yes, my days are numbered and I have numbered them according to my wishes, decisions and deeds. And when these grey, dull days draw to a close, I shall laugh at the dreams I have dreamt; and I shall slam this earthly door behind me as my flight to eternity begins.

S.Y.

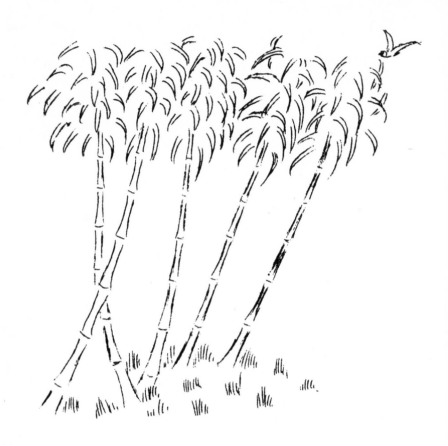

Each part is like the whole: everything springs from the whole, from God.

Vivekananda

Stand at a point of vantage: knowing our universal nature, we must look with perfect calmness upon the whole panorama of the world.

V.

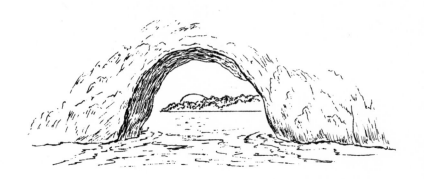

A zealous adherent of the maharshi was troubled because
somebody in the town had spoken disparagingly of the
master and he had not answered him back. He asked the
master what the penalty for this omission was.

M: Patience, and more patience! Tolerance—and more
   tolerance.

Sri Ramana Maharshi

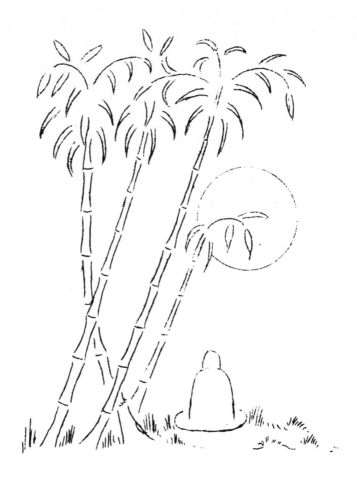

Do you know how I see God? I see him as all and everything. Man and other creatures seem to me to be empty
husks which move their heads and limbs but their content
is God.

Ramakrishna

If we have the three greatest 'gifts of God': a human body,
the ardent wish to be free, and the help of someone who
has achieved that aim and can show us the way, then our
liberation is certain.

Vivekananda

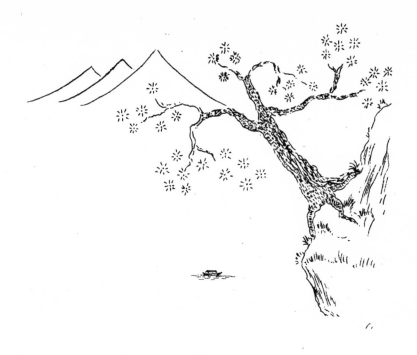

'This SELF is first to be heard of.' Hear day and night
that you are that SELF. Repeat it to yourself day and night
until it enters into your very veins, until it tingles in every
drop of blood, until it is in your flesh and bone. Let the
whole body be full of that one ideal, 'I am the birthless,
the deathless, the blissful, the omniscient, the omnipotent,
ever-glorious SELF'. All your actions will be magnified,
transformed, deified, by the very power of the thought.
If matter is mighty, thought is almighty.

Vivekananda

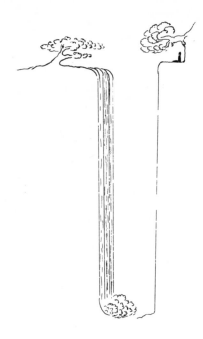

There is, O monks, an unborn, an unbecome, an unmade, an uncompounded; if, monks, there were not here this unborn, unbecome, unmade, uncompounded, there would not here be an escape from the born, the become, the made, the compounded. But because there is an unborn, an unbecome, an unmade, an uncompounded, therefore, there is an escape from the born, the become, the made, the compounded.

Buddha

That which is Infinite is truly happiness; there is no happiness in the finite; the Infinite alone is happiness. One should therefore seek to know the Infinite alone.

Upanishad

36

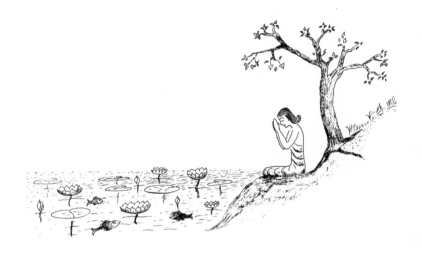

Decadence seizes everything in this life. It is only when everything, even love, fails, that, with a flash, man finds out how vain, how dreamlike is this world. Then he catches a glimpse of renunciation, catches a glimpse of the Beyond. It is only by giving up this world that the other comes; never through holding on to this one. The cause of misery is the clash between the different forces of nature, one dragging one way, and another dragging another, rendering permanent happiness impossible. Never yet was there a great soul who had not to reject sense pleasures and enjoyments to acquire his greatness.

Vivekananda

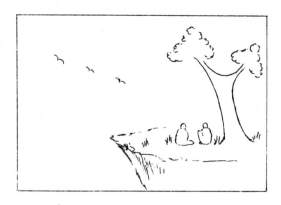

We live happily indeed, not hating those who hate us!
Among men who hate us we dwell free from hatred!

Good men are seen from afar, like the snowy mountains;
bad people are not seen, like arrows shot in the night.

He who holds back rising anger like a rolling chariot, him
I call a real driver; other people are but holding the reins.

Buddha

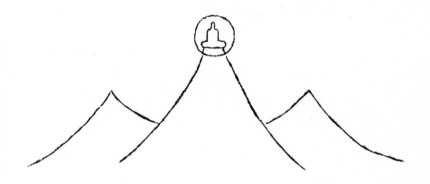

Rest assured that if you serve TRUTH in spite of tempta-
tions to forsake it, you will attain a heavenly strength, in
the face of which men will quail to speak before you
things which you do not believe to be true. People will
be convinced by what you say to them if you can strictly
serve TRUTH for fourteen years continually without
swerving from it. Thus you will confer the greatest blessing
on the masses, unshackle their bondages and uplift the
whole nation.

Vivekananda

Man! What a mighty thought!
Projected by the infinite
To watch the play of life and death;
To create fates
And whirl destinies into space,
And laugh as they burst as rockets,
Casting their ashes upon the shores
Of forgotten worlds.

                                        S.Y.

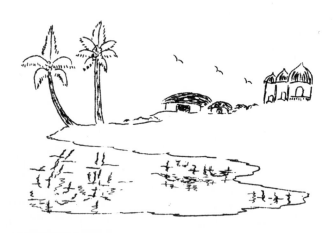

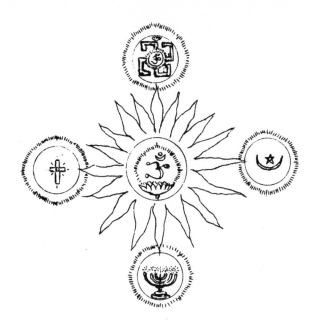

Bring all light into the world. Light, bring light! Let light come unto everyone; the task will not be finished till everyone has reached the Lord. Bring light to the poor, and bring more light to the rich, for they require it more than the poor. Bring light to the ignorant, and more light to the educated, for the vanities of the education of our time are tremendous! Thus bring light to all.

Vivekananda

Spirituality must be brought to the practical level of life. Otherwise what use is it? Spirituality must uplift the heart and the home, the individual and the crowd, society and the nation.

S.Y.

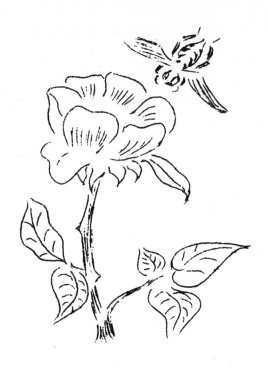

Ye divinities on earth! Sinners? It is a sin to call a man so; it is a standing libel on human nature. Come up O lions, and shake off the delusion that you are sheep; you are souls immortal, spirits free, blessed and eternal; ye are not matter, ye are not bodies; matter is your servant, not you the servants of matter.

Vivekananda

Be thou the pioneer of thine own path
and tread with boldness every measured step.
With an unbending will, launch into deeds
The demands of thine only guide,
Thy god, thy very Self.

S.Y.

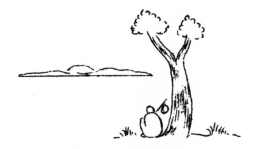

D: The world is materialistic. What is the remedy for it?

M: Materialistic or spiritual, it is according to your outlook. Make your outlook right. The Creator knows how to take care of His Creation.

D: What is the best thing to do for ensuring the future?

M: Take care of the present, the future will take care of itself.

As you are, so is the world. Without understanding yourself, what is the use of trying to understand the world? This is a question that seekers after truth need not consider. People waste their energies over all such questions. First, find out the truth behind yourself; then you will be in a better position to understand the truth behind the world, of which you are a part.

M.

The life of action need not be renounced. If you will meditate for an hour or two every day, you can then carry on with your duties. If you meditate in the right manner, then the current of mind induced will continue to flow even in the midst of your work. It is as though there were two ways of expressing the same idea; the line which you take in meditation will be expressed in your activities. As you go on you will find that your attitude towards people, events and objects will gradually change. Your actions will tend to follow your meditations of their own accord.

M.

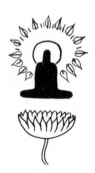

You are blessed indeed! You are drawing near to the goal. Through you, your whole family have become purified, because you long to get free from the bondage of ignorance and reach Brahman (GOD).

Know, O wise one, that man needs freedom from passion and the power of discrimination as the bird needs its two wings. Without these man can never reach the highest grape from which the nectar of freedom flows.

Sankaracharya

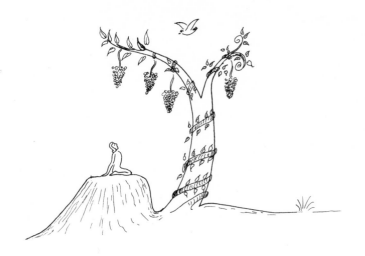

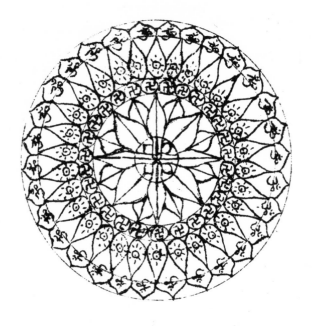

Ye are the light of the world. A city that is set on a hill cannot be hid. Neither do men light a candle, and put it under a bushel, but on a candlestick; and it giveth light unto all that are in the house. Let your light so shine before men, that they may see your good works, and glorify your Father which is in heaven.

Matthew 5, v. 14–16

46

Even the greatest sinner, who has sinned during one hundred incarnations, will be freed from all sin if he can realise his divine being, be it but for half a second. He will be pure, perfect, and divine still in this life.

Vedanta Phil.

Do you know the true meaning of the word Buddha? It means that by constantly thinking about consciousness one becomes consciousness itself.

Ramakrishna

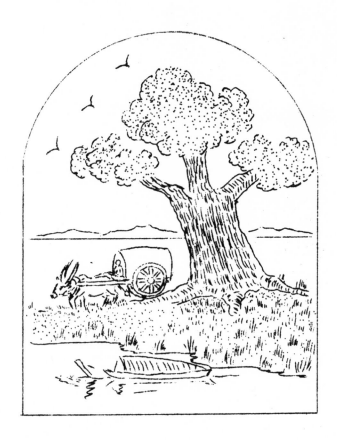

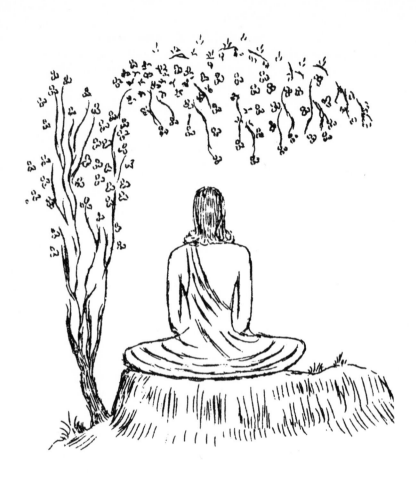

It is not possible to pray to the Absolute but only to a manifestation of the Absolute. Jesus had the nature of man. He became Christ. We too can and *must* do that. Christ and Buddha are the names for a state that is to be achieved. Jesus and Gautama were the figures that manifested the state.

Vivekananda

Rise, thou radiant one! Rise, thou eternally pure one! Rise, thou who wert never born and canst never die. Rise, thou almighty one. Manifest thy true nature. These lowly manifestations are unworthy of thee.

A man who has purified himself to the uttermost achieves more than a whole regiment of preachers. The word of power comes from purity and silence.

Vivekananda

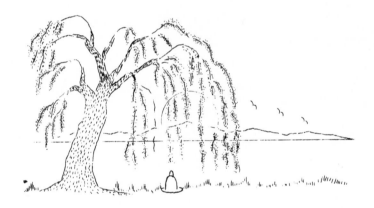

The greatest of all men uses his heart like a mirror. He does not seek things and does not go out to them; he reflects them but does not perpetuate their image. Thus he can conquer the world and is not wounded. He is not the slave of his reputation; he hatches no plans; he has nothing to do with business; he is the master of knowledge. He takes heed of the smallest things and is yet inexhaustible and tarries the far side of self. He accepts to the last iota what heaven gives, and yet it is as if he had nothing. He remains humble.

Tchuang Dsi

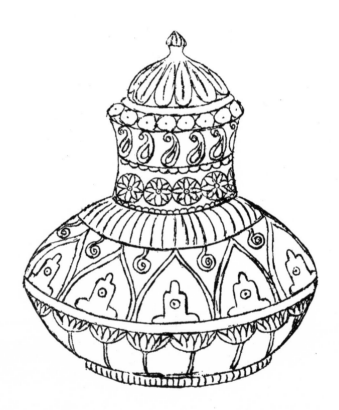

Where art Thou to be found, O my Maker?
Where art Thou to be seen, O my Lord?
In the worship hour of dawn should I seek Thee?
In the vesperal hour of even art Thou here?

Where the fire-fly lights up the path of the forest,
Where the babbling brook sings her ceaseless songs,
Where the blades of bright lightning fall on earth's bosom,
Where the thundering clouds pour down their rain,
Where death's touch has brought hope for the departed,
Where the birth of a babe brings sunshine to all,
There Thou art, O Lord, in my worship,
There Thou art from dawn till eventide.

S.Y.

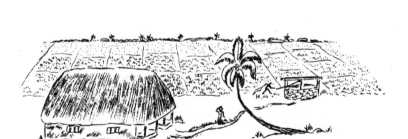

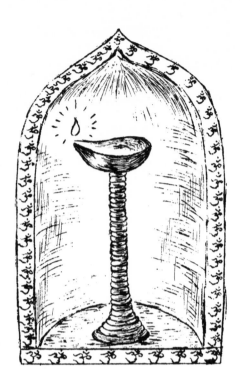

Nothing we do is ever lost in all eternity.
As time unfolds all things bear fruit in their maturity.
Suffering is the most disliked teacher who in hours of loneliness teaches us the lessons we need.

S.Y.

The man who accepts gifts is spiritually under the influence of the giver, and in this way the recipient can be influenced. Accepting gifts means surrendering our spiritual independence and enslaving ourselves. Therefore do not accept gifts.

Vivekananda

Man is shaped by circumstances, and it is he himself who causes them.

S.Y.

WHAT IS GOD?

He who lives in the earth—and yet is different from the earth—whom the earth does not know—whose body is the earth, who governs the earth inwardly—HE is thy SELF, THINE INNER guide, thine immortal part.

He who lives in heaven—and yet is different from heaven—whom heaven does not know—whose body is heaven—who governs heaven inwardly—HE is thy SELF, thine inner guide, thine immortal part.

He who lives in the light—and yet is different from the light—whom the light does not know—whose body is the light—who governs the light inwardly—HE is thy SELF, thine inner guide, thine immortal part.

He who lives in breath—and yet is different from breath—whom breath does not know—whose body is breath—who governs breath inwardly—HE is thy SELF, thine inner guide, thine immortal part.

He who lives in thought—and yet differs from thought—whom thought does not know—whose body is thought—who governs thinking inwardly—HE is thy SELF, thine inner guide, thine immortal part.

He who lives in knowledge—and yet differs from knowledge—whom knowledge does not know—whose body is knowledge, who governs knowledge inwardly—HE is thy SELF, thine inner guide, thine immortal part.

HE is seeing—not seen—hearing—not heard—understanding—not understood—knowing—not known; apart from HIM there is none that sees—none that hears—none that understands—none that knows—HE is thy SELF, thine inner guide, thine IMMORTAL PART!

Upanishads

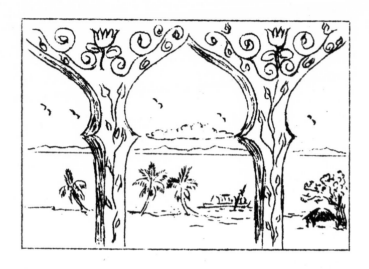

A father had two sons. When they reached the right age, they were admitted into the class of those seeking initiation (brahmacharya) and placed in the care of a religious teacher to study the Vedas.

After a long absence the boys returned home on completing their studies. Their father asked them whether they had read the Vedanta. When they replied that they had, he asked: 'What is Brahman?' (God).

The eldest, who quoted the Vedas and other holy writings, replied: 'O Father, it cannot be conceived through the spoken word or the power of the understanding. O, it is thus and thus. I know all about it.' He then began to quote Vedic texts.

The father said: 'I see you have recognised Brahman! You may go to your work.' Then he asked the younger son the same question. But the boy sat quite dumb. He neither said a word nor made the slightest attempt to speak.

Then the father said: 'Nothing can be said about the Absolute and Unconditional! No sooner do you speak of it than you define the Infinite with concepts of the finite, the Absolute with concepts of the relative, the Unconditional with concepts of the conditional. Thy silence is more eloquent than the repetition of hundreds of verses and the quotation of hundreds of authorities.'

Ramakrishna

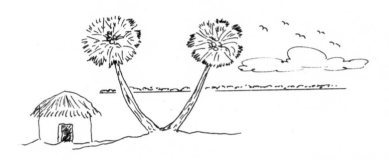

An angler caught fish in a pool. The Avadhuta (mendicant monk) approached and asked: 'Brother, which is the path to such and such a place?' Just then the float indicated that a fish was nibbling at the bait. And so the man did not reply but concentrated on the fishing rod. When the fish was caught, he turned round and said: 'What did you say, Sir?' The monk bowed to him and said: 'Sir, be my guru (spiritual teacher). When I am absorbed in contemplation of the Highest Self, let me follow your example and pay heed to nothing else until my meditation is ended!'

Ramakrishna

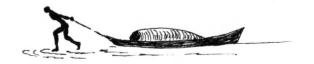

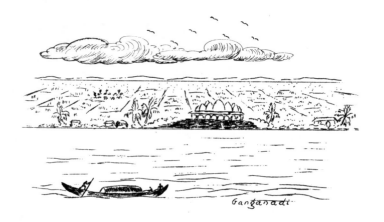

Gangānadī

Go into yourself and bring the Upanishads out of your own self. You are the greatest book that ever was and ever will be, the infinite treasury of everything that is. All external teaching is in vain unless the inner teacher is awake. It must lead to the opening of the book of the heart to have any value.

Vivekananda

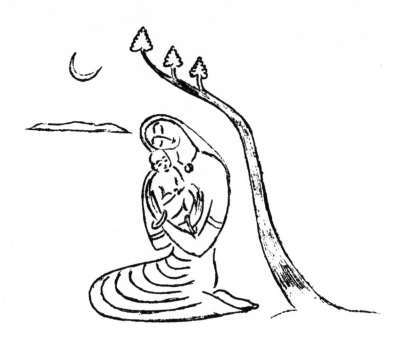

And may my song to you, my love, carry you
    to the limitless land of my dreams.
And with the unseen wings of night may you
    fly from star to star.
And beyond the borders of sleep may you
    wander many a world.
And on the golden streaks of dawn
    come back to mother's arms,
Where the matchless beauty of the morn
    awaits to open your eyes, my love.

S.Y.

Life is growth and expansion. The goal of human life is to express the divinity we potentially are. The expression of our infinite and universal nature is the great struggle of life.

Suffering must always be considered in a positive light, for without it there can be no growth. We should regard suffering as our growing pains.

S.Y.

As long as we still have the feeling of sympathy, we are not free. We are not free from 'antipathy'. True love transcends sympathy and antipathy.

S.Y.

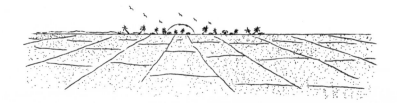

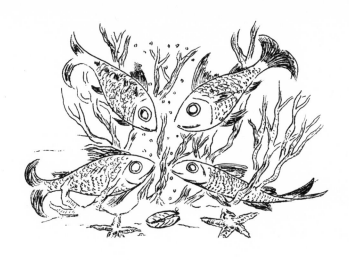

Spirituality has nothing to do with sentimentality. Nor does spirituality allow an attitude of indifference in an unhealthy or unacceptable situation. The truthful man knows no compromises. Be honest, open and free, as each given situation requires.

S.Y.

Activity properly refrained from brings freedom.
Activity properly carried out brings freedom.
Both are better than the shunning of activity.

Bhagavad Gita

Disburden your ship of passions and hate, O sailor, and you will sail lightly to freedom.

Elisabeth Haich

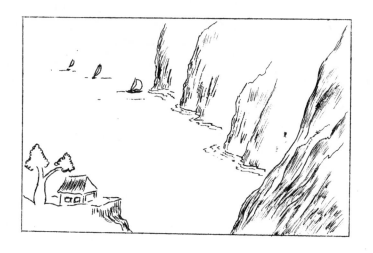

Your own will is all that answers prayer, but it appears under the guise of different religious conceptions to each mind. We may call it Buddha, Jesus, Krishna, Jehovah, Allah, Agni, but it is only the Self, the 'I'.

Vivekananda

What great bliss it is to be able to partake of divine growth! Think back into your past and compare it with your present, and you will realise the long process of development you have passed through. All our true knowledge is based on our own experience. Inward progress alone makes man happy.

S.Y.

D: How can I control the mind?
M: There is no mind to control if the Self is realised.

Sri Ramana Maharshi

The strength of a nation lies not in its army of soldiers but in its men of morals. A few such will suffice to awaken the real character of the people, by the sheer force of their example. And what is stronger than character?

S.Y.

What we want is a religion that forms men! We need men!
Men with muscles of iron and nerves of steel.

Vivekananda

It is not love that is blind but lust. Men are blinded by sensual desires. Real love liberates a man from lust.

S.Y.

Be fearless and strong. The world esteems only its heroes.

S.Y.

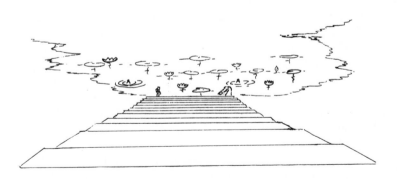

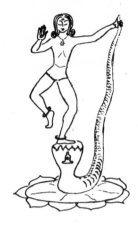

Krishna's dance on the five-headed serpent. Mastery of the spirit over the five senses.

Honour both spirit and material form; the inherent thought as well as the visible symbol.

Sri Ramakrishna

At the centre of every existing religion there is a great teacher who preaches the truth; the masses follow him. Without the teacher the religious edifice decays. The Vedas are the only sacred doctrines which are not based on a particular personality or scripture but establish man as such at the centre of evolution and raise him to the ultimate level of divinity. Their laws are all-embracing and guide man's inner development. The Vedas bring out man's innermost being—irrespective of the creed he embraces—and help him to realise his aim. Therefore they are held to be a universal religion which raises up a man within his own particular faith.

S.Y.

He who can transform his animal forces into spiritual powers becomes a storehouse of strength. All progress is based on the control of the animal forces within. Let them loose, and they mercilessly drag you down. Harness them, and they make gods out of men.

S.Y.

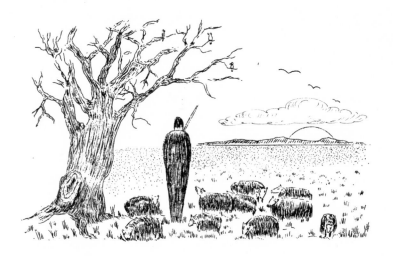

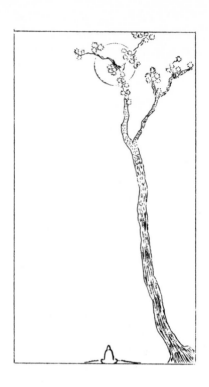

Who is blind? He who takes pleasure in what he may not
do.
Who is deaf? He who does not hear salutary words.
Who is dumb? He who can say nothing kind at the right
time.

Indian proverb

If one has succeeded in being born a human being, it
would be a pity to ruin this human life by senseless or
wicked actions and then to end a wretched existence by
death.

Tagpo Lhadje

An honest thought can move heaven and earth.

Chinese proverb

The quality of forbearance is of the highest importance to every man. He alone is not destroyed, who possesses this quality.

When an elephant is let loose it goes about uprooting trees and shrubs, but as soon as the keeper pricks him on the head with a goad, he becomes quiet; so the mind, when unrestrained, wantons in the luxuriance of idle thoughts, but becomes at once calm when struck with the goad of right discrimination.

He alone enters the kingdom of heaven who is not a thief of his own thoughts. In other words, guilelessness and simple faith are the road to that kingdom.

Sri Ramakrishna

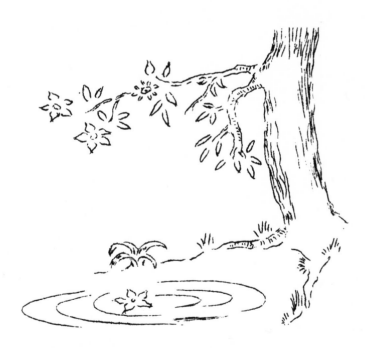

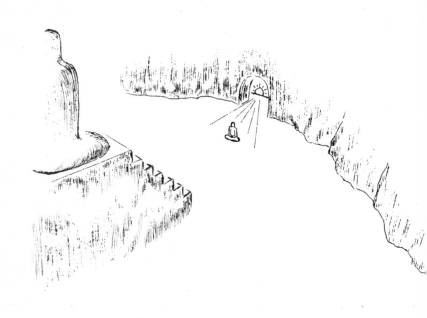

The eternal flicker of this lamp doth glow and shine.
Sunk in the depths of silence,
What matters else but to know that
'I AM'

S.Y.

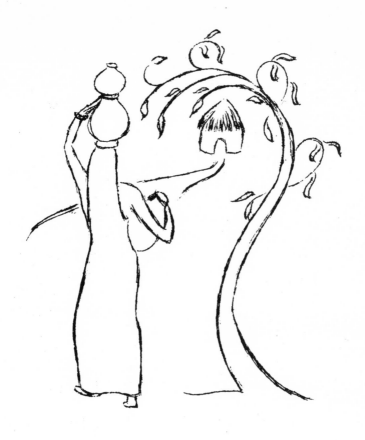

In spiritual matters your thought should be just as rational as in everyday affairs. External affairs call for rational thought. The spiritual life calls for a thousandfold measure of rational, precise, well-founded thought.

S.Y.

Prayer is a wonderful aid, for it is the only opportunity of really helping oneself.

S.Y.

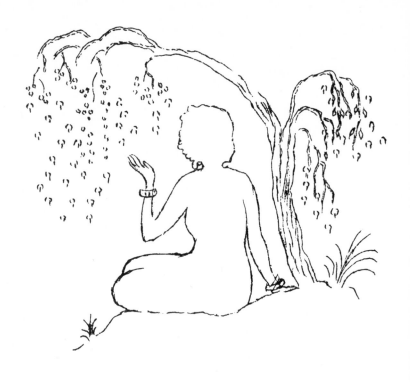

Which is the path to Heaven?
Truthfulness.

How does a man find happiness?
Through correct conduct.

What must he subdue in order to avoid sorrow?
His thoughts.

When is a man loved?
When he is without vanity.

Mahabharata

The Self is not only the easiest thing to know, but beyond It there is nothing else to know. All that is required to realise the Self is TO BE STILL. And what can be easier than that?

Bhagavan Ramana Maharshi

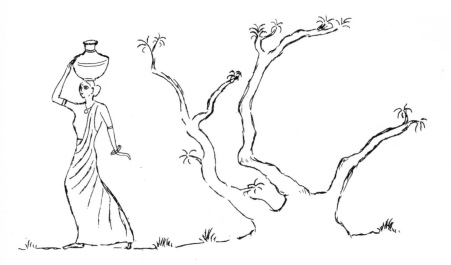

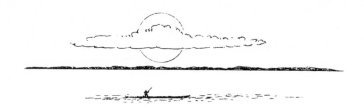

Try to understand that you are spiritual only when you begin to recognise God in man, when you grasp that you are the spirit that pervades all: the bright crystal, the smiling flower, the dumb animal, the thinking man.

S.Y.

No one is born so lowly that he cannot rise. He who rises emerges from the depths.

S.Y.

Only by the wave falling back into the sea can it become unlimited, never as a wave can it be so. Then after it has become the sea, it can become the wave again and as big a one as it pleases. Break the identification of yourself with the current and know that you are free.

Vivekananda

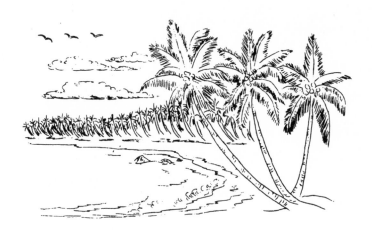

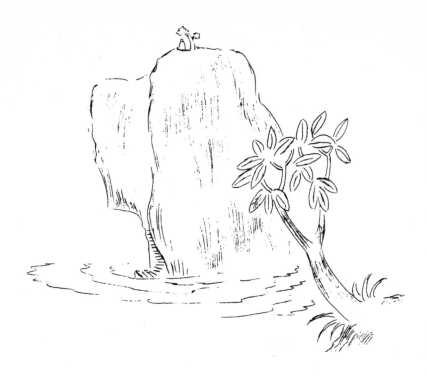

There is, however, one impurity that exceeds all impurities—and that is ignorance. O wise one, cast off that impurity and be free from all impurities.

Dhammapada

He who heeds not the evil report of others vanquishes all.

Mahabharata

Between him that performeth without fatigue sacrifices every month for a hundred years and him that never feeleth angry at anything, he that feeleth not wrath is certainly the higher.

Mahabharata

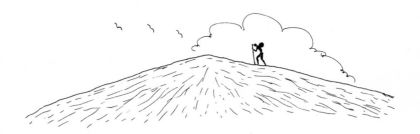

Ignorant am I of the ways of the world, and I know not what to do. Guide my steps to do right, never faltering for fear or shame.

S.Y.

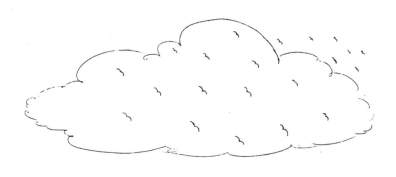

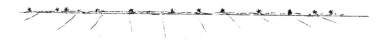

Disciple: Is solitude helpful for practice?

Maharshi: What do you mean by solitude?

Disciple: To keep away from others.

Maharshi: What is the good of that? It is actuated only
by fear and uncertainty. Even in solitude there is the
fear of intrusion by others and of solitude being spoilt.
Moreover, how are thoughts to be erased in solitude?
Can it not be done equally well in your present
environment.

Sri Ramana Maharshi

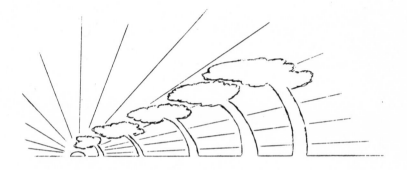

He is a truly spiritual man who has an unshakable faith in himself and is capable of realising this even in his simplest thoughts and daily actions.

S.Y.

You are free and not free at the same time—never free on the earthly plane, but ever free on the spiritual. Go beyond both freedom and bondage.

Say it is your 'nature' to do it; never say it is your 'duty' to do anything whatever.

Vivekananda

3 Yoga Exercises through the Year

A FEW VITAL POINTS TO REMEMBER

1. Start the day with Yoga, devoting at least 30 to 40 min to practice.
2. With this perseverance, the three great blessings of life, Health, Wealth and Happiness, will be yours.
3. Regular practice is most important, for the latent forces of the body are thus liberated and made to unfold and become manifest as WILL-POWER, POWER OF CONCENTRATION, POWER OF DETERMINATION, POWER OF RESISTANCE, etc., affording natural immunity to illness and harmful influences.
4. The mantrams form an indispensable part of the training. Repetition of all of them, or even a few chosen suggestions, during the daily practice of Yoga is important. They will enter and take root in the subconscious mind, and will compel the body to obey and fulfil the demands of the spirit. 'The body is the outer covering of the mind. Whatever the mind dictates, the body has to obey. . . . If matter is mighty, thought is almighty!'
5. As the empty stomach receives food and assimilates it, so the subconscious mind receives these good impressions and brings forth in time admirable traits of character such as fearlessness, courage, steadfastness, strong will, and an ever-growing sense of freedom.
6. The mental repetition of mantrams is warmly recommended just before falling asleep. The current of the mind thus induced will continue even during sleep and foster a healthy and positive outlook on life.
7. 'The body is the chariot, the five senses the steeds, the mind the reins, but I AM THE CHARIOTEER!' Maintain this attitude, steer your own destiny, and BE FREE.

Mantrams: My power of resistance is growing from moment to moment.

My will-power is growing from moment to moment.

Every organ is working better and better from
moment to moment.
I manifest life in the body and the mind.
Rest and peace.
OM—OM—OM.

Week 1

1. Abdominal, middle, upper, and complete Yoga breathing (Rest) — 7 × each

2. Jalandhara-Bandha (Retain breath for 7–30 sec with chin pressing against the chest) Will-power — 3 ×

3. Chest tapping (During inhalation tap the chest rapidly with the fingertips. Retain breath and slap quickly with the palms of the hands) Purity — 3 ×

4. Development of solar energy — 3 min

5. Abdominal and leg muscle exercise — 3 ×

6. Bhujangendrasana (Strong nerves) — 3 ×

7. Matsyasana (Rest) — 3 ×

8. Exercise for the small of the back — 3 ×

9. Hastapadangustasana (Stability) — 3 ×

10. Lauliki-Yoga (Inhale, protrude abdomen, exhale, press the abdomen hard with the palms from left to right) — 3 × 7 ×

11. Ardha-Halasana (Elasticity) — 3 ×

12. Sirshasana (Rejuvenation) — 3 ×

13. Meditation (Unity) — 5 min

14. Savasana (Perfect relaxation) — 5 min

OM

Week 2

1. Abdominal, middle, upper, and complete Yoga breathing (Rest)   7 × each

2. Jalandhara-Bandha (Retain breath for 7–30 sec with chin pressing against the chest) Will-power   3 ×

3. Sukh-purvak (Alternate breathing right and left) Purity   3 ×

4. Sitkari (Breathe in between tip of tongue and palate) Blood cleansing   10 ×

5. Yoga-Mudra (With fist on abdomen) Health   3 ×

6. Ardha-Matsyendrasana (Strong nerves)   3 ×

7. Janusirasana I (Resistance)   3 ×

8. Janusirasana II (Resistance)   3 ×

9. Bhegasana (Elasticity)   3 ×

10. Gokarnasana (Figure and beauty)   3 ×

11. Natarajasana (Figure and beauty)   3 ×

12. Viparita-Karani (With exercises to strengthen the eyes) Rejuvenation   3 ×

13. Meditation (Unity)   5 min

14. Savasana (Perfect relaxation)   5 min

OM

Week 3

1. Abdominal, middle, upper, and complete Yoga breathing (Rest) — 7 × each

2. Jalandhara-Bandha (Retain breath for 7–30 sec with chin pressing against the chest) Will-power — 3 ×

3. Bhastrika (Accelerated complete breathing) Purity — 10 ×

4. Sitali (Inhale through the tube-formed tongue) Blood purification — 14 ×

5. Pavanamuktasana (Clasp the knees tightly) Health — 3 × 7 ×

6. Bhujangendrasana (Strong nerves) — 3 ×

7. Janusirasana horizontal (Resistance) — 3 ×

8. Janusirasana vertical (Resistance) — 3 ×

9. Dolasana (Figure and beauty) — 3 ×

10. Natashira Vajrasana (Strength) — 3 ×

11. Vajroli-Mudra (Strength) — 3 ×

12. Ardha-Sarvangsana (Rejuvenation) — 5 min

13. Meditation (Unity) — 5 min

14. Savasana (Perfect relaxation) — 5 min

OM

Week 4

1. Abdominal, middle, upper, and complete Yoga breathing (Rest)   7 × each

2. Jalandhara-Bandha (Retain breath for 7–30 sec with chin pressing against chest) Will-power   3 ×

3. Chest tapping (During inhalation tap the chest rapidly with the fingertips. Retain breath and slap quickly with the palms of the hands) Purity   3 ×

4. Cleansing breathing   3 ×

5. Ustrasana (Elasticity)   3 ×

6. Paschimotanasana (Health)   3 ×

7. Ardha-Matsyendrasana II (Self-confidence)   3 ×

8. Trikonasana (I am straight in body and mind)   3 ×

9. Trikonasana   3 ×

10. Bend forward with the legs wide apart, palms, elbows and head on the floor. Breathe quietly (Stand up again after 7–10 sec) Complete relaxation   3 ×

11. Vrksasana (Equilibrium)   3 ×

12. Halasana (Elasticity)   3 ×

13. Meditation (Unity)   5 min

14. Savasana (Perfect relaxation)   5 min

OM

Week 5

1. Abdominal, middle, upper, and complete Yoga breathing (Rest) — 7 × each

2. Jalandhara-Bandha (Retain breath for 7–14 sec with chin pressing against chest) Will-power — 3 ×

3. Cleansing breathing (Seated) — 3 ×

4. 'S' breathing (Seated) Purity — 3 ×

5. Vakrasana (Strong nerves) — 3 ×

6. Yoga-Mudra (With fist on abdomen) Health — 3 ×

7. Bhujangasana (Strong nerves) — 3 ×

8. Ardha-Salabhasana (Kidneys) Purity — 3 ×

9. Trikonasana (Strong nerves) — 3 ×

10. Uddiyana-Bandha (Draw abdomen in tight) Resistance — 3 ×

11. Uddiyana-Bandha (Standing) Resistance — 3 ×

12. Viparita-Karani (Rejuvenation) — 3 ×

13. Meditation (Unity) — 5 min

14. Savasana (Perfect relaxation) — 5 min

OM

Week 6

1. Abdominal, middle, upper, and complete Yoga breathing (Rest) — 7 × each

2. Jalandhara-Bandha (Retain breath for 7–30 sec with chin pressing against chest) Will-power — 3 ×

3. Ha-breathing (Lying: slow) Purity — 3 ×

4. Ha-breathing (Standing: slow) Purity — 3 ×

5. Bhujangasana (Kidneys) Purity — 3 ×

6. Bhujangendrasana (Spine) Strength — 3 ×

7. Maha-Mudra (Resistance) — 3 ×

8. Vakrasana (Strong nerves) — 3 ×

9. Tadaghi-Mudra (Draw abdomen in tight) Resistance — 3 ×

10. Dolasana (Spine) Elasticity — 3 ×

11. Ardha-Chandrasana (Elasticity) — 3 ×

12. Sarvangasana (Thyroid) Rejuvenation — 3 ×

13. Meditation (Unity) — 5 min

14. Savasana (Perfect relaxation) — 5 min

OM

Week 7

1. Abdominal, middle, upper, and complete Yoga breathing (Rest)   7 × each

2. Jalandhara-Bandha (Retain breath for 7–14 sec with chin pressing against chest) Will-power   3 ×

3. Ha-breathing (Lying: vigorously) Purity   3 ×

4. Bhastrika (Bellows-breathing) Purity   3 ×

5. Yoga-Mudra (Health)   3 ×

6. Padahastasana (Resistance)   3 ×

7. Bhujangasana (Strong nerves)   3 ×

8. Vakrasana (Strong nerves)   3 ×

9. Janusirasana (Resistance)   3 ×

10. Ekapadahastasana I (Figure and beauty)   2 ×

11. Ekapadahastasana II (Figure and beauty)   2 ×

12. Viparita-Karani (Rejuvenation)   3 ×

13. Meditation (Unity)   5 min

14. Savasana (Perfect relaxation)   5 min

OM

85

Week 8

1. Abdominal, middle, upper, and complete Yoga breathing (Prana body development) 7 × each

2. Inhale deeply and then empty the lungs, tense chest and abdominal muscles, retain breath for 7 sec. Inhale deeply (Resistance) 3 ×

3. Sukh-purvak (Equilibrium and harmony) 3 ×

4. Bhastrika (Bellows-breathing) Purity 3 ×

5. Parshva-Bhunamanasana (Resistance) 3 ×

6. Vakrasana (Strong nerves) 3 ×

7. Ardha-Matsyendrasana (Strong nerves) 3 ×

8. Kaakaasana (Raven posture) Equilibrium 3 ×

9. Dolasana (Figure and beauty) 3 ×

10. Ardha-Bhujangasana I and II (Strong nerves) 2 × each

11. Salabhasana (Kidneys) Purity 3 ×

12. Sarvangasana (Rejuvenation) 3 ×

13. Meditation (Unity) 5 min

14. Savasana (Perfect relaxation) 5 min

OM

Week 9

1. Abdominal, middle, upper, and complete Yoga breathing (Rest) — 7 × each

2. Jalandhara-Bandha (Retain breath for 7–30 sec with chin pressing against chest) Will-power — 3 ×

3. Pranayama No. 1 (Resistance) — 3 ×

4. Chest-tapping exercise (Slowly inhale, rapidly tapping the chest with the finger-tips. Retain breath and slap the chest with the palms) Lung cleansing — 3 ×

5. Vakrasana (Strong nerves) — 2 ×

6. Vakrasana (Variation) Strong nerves — 2 ×

7. Ardha-Bhujangasana — 3° ×

8. Parshva-Bhunamanasana (Elasticity) — 3 ×

9. Uddiyana-Bandha (Standing) Self-control — 3 ×

10. Natapadasana (Strength) — 3 ×

11. Foot exercises — 3 min

12. Sirshasana or Viparita-Karani (Rejuvenation) — 3 ×

13. Meditation (Unity) — 5 min

14. Savasana (Perfect relaxation) — 5 min

OM

Week 10

1. Abdominal, middle, upper, and complete Yoga breathing (Rest) 7 × each

2. Jalandhara-Bandha (Retain breath for 7–30 sec with chin pressing against chest) Will-power 3 ×

3. 'S' Breathing (Purity) 3 ×

4. I.A.O.OM 3 ×

5. Stambhasana (Resistance) 3 ×

6. Bhujangendrasana (Spine) Strength 3 ×

7. Ardha-Salabhasana (Kidneys) Purity 2 ×

8. Salabhasana (Kidneys) Purity 3 ×

9. Yoga-Mudra (Lift arms vertically) Health 3 ×

10. Padahastasana (Health) 3 ×

11. Uddiyana-Bandha (Standing) Self-control 3 ×

12. Sirshasana or Halasana (Rejuvenation) 3 ×

13. Meditation (Unity) 5 min

14. Savasana (Perfect relaxation) 5 min

OM

Week 11

1. Abdominal, middle, upper, and complete Yoga breathing (Rest)   7 × each

2. Jalandhara-Bandha (Retain breath for 7–30 sec with chin pressing against the chest) Will-power   3 ×

3. Chest tapping (During inhalation tap the chest rapidly with the fingertips. Retain breath and slap chest with the palms) Purity   3 ×

4. Sitali (Inhale through tube-formed tongue) Blood cleansing   3 × 9 ×

5. Trikonasana (I am straight in body and in mind)   3 ×

6. Trikonasana (Variation) Strong nerves   3 ×

7. Pavanamuktasana lying (Clasp knees tightly) Health   3 × 9 ×

8. Lauliki-Yoga (Health)   3 ×

9. Ardha-Bhujangasana   3 ×

10. Ardha-Salabhasana (Kidneys) Purity   3 ×

11. Ustrasana (Elasticity)   3 ×

12. Viparita-Karani (With exercises to strengthen the eyes) Rejuvenation   3 ×

13. Meditation (Unity)   5 min

14. Savasana (Perfect relaxation)   5 min

OM

Week 12

1. Abdominal, middle, upper, and complete Yoga breathing (Rest) — 7 × each

2. Jalandhara-Bandha (Retain breath for 7–30 sec with chin pressing against the chest) Will-power — 3 ×

3. Ha-breathing (Lying: slowly) Purity — 3 ×

4. Ha-breathing (Standing: slowly) Purity — 3 ×

5. Dhrityasana (Stability) — 3 ×

6. Dhanurasana (Elasticity) — 3 ×

7. Bhujangasana (Strong nerves) — 3 ×

8. Vakrasana (Strong nerves) — 3 ×

9. Ekapadahastasana I and II (Figure and beauty) — 2 × each

10. Janusirasana (Vertical) Figure and beauty — 2 ×

11. Janusirasana (Horizontal) Figure and beauty — 2 ×

12. Halasana (Legs apart) Elasticity — 3 ×

13. Meditation (Unity) — 5 min

14. Savasana (Perfect relaxation) — 5 min

OM

Week 13

1. Abdominal, middle, upper, and complete Yoga breathing (Rest) — 7 × each

2. Jalandhara-Bandha (Retain breath for 7–30 sec with chin pressing against the chest) Will-power — 3 ×

3. Sukh-purvak (4–16–8 sec) Alternating breathing harmony — 5 ×

4. Pranayama No. 4 (Strength) — 3 ×

5. Chakrasana (Wheel posture) Elasticity — 3 ×

6. Dhrityasana (Resolution) — 3 ×

7. Paschimotanasana (Health) — 3 ×

8. Supta-Vajrasana (Charging of solar plexus) — 3 ×

9. Mayurasana (Equilibrium) — 3 ×

10. Gokarnasana (Figure and beauty) — 3 ×

11. Hastapadasana (Legs wide apart. Hold toes and then bend forward while exhaling) — 3 ×

12. Sirshasana (Rejuvenation) — 3 ×

13. Viparita-Karani (Rejuvenation) — 3 ×

14. Meditation (Unity) — 5 min

15. Savasana (Perfect relaxation) — 5 min

OM

Week 14

1. Abdominal, middle, upper, and complete Yoga breathing (Rest) — 7 × each

2. Jalandhara-Bandha (Retain breath for 7–10 sec with chin pressing against the chest) Will-power — 3 ×

3. Pranayama No. 3 — 3 ×

4. Pranayama No. 4 (Strength) — 3 ×

5. Lauliki-Mudra (Abdominal massage) — 3 ×

6. Yoga-Mudra (With fist on abdomen) Health — 3 ×

7. Vajroli-Mudra (Resistance) — 3 ×

8. Bhujangasana (Strong nerves) — 3 ×

9. Salabhasana (Kidneys) Purity — 3 ×

10. Matsyasana (Rest) — 3 ×

11. Eye-strengthening exercises (Bru-Madya-Drishti: fixation between the eyebrows. Nasagra-Drishti: fixation of nose tip) — 3 ×

12. Sarvangasana (Rejuvenation) — 3 ×

13. Meditation (Unity) — 5 min

14. Savasana (Perfect relaxation) — 5 min

OM

Week 15

1. Abdominal, middle, upper, and complete Yoga breathing (Prana body development)   7 × each

2. Jalandhara-Bandha (Retain breath for 7–30 sec with chin pressing against the chest) Will-power   3 ×

3. Pranayama No. 6   3 ×

4. Pranayama No. 7   3 ×

5. Vibhakta-Janusirasana (Resistance)   3 ×

6. Natashira-Vajrasana (Strength)   3 ×

7. Janusirasana (Vertical) Resistance   2 ×

8. Janusirasana (Horizontal) Resistance   2 ×

9. Dolasana (Elasticity)   3 ×

10. Lauliki-Yoga (Abdominal massage)   3 ×

11. Foot exercises   3 min

12. Viparita-Karani (With tongue exercise) Rejuvenation   3 ×

13. Meditation (Unity)   5 min

14. Savasana (Perfect relaxation)   5 min

OM

Week 16

1. Abdominal, middle, upper, and complete Yoga breathing (Prana body development)   7 × each

2. Jalandhara-Bandha (Retain breath for 7–30 sec with chin pressing against the chest) Will-power   3 ×

3. Ha-breathing (Lying: vigorously) Purity   3 ×

4. Pranayama No. 4 (Strength)   3 ×

5. Vakrasana (Strong nerves)   3 ×

6. Trikonasana (Variation) Strong nerves   3 ×

7. Trikonasana (Variation) I am straight in body and mind   3 ×

8. Mantrams:
   My power of resistance is growing from moment to moment.
   My will-power is growing from moment to moment.
   Every organ is working better and better from moment to moment.
   I manifest life in the body and the mind.
   Rest and peace.   3 × each
   OM—OM—OM

9. Pavanamuktasana (Clasp the knees tightly) Health   3 × 9 ×

10. Natapadasana (Strength)   3 ×

11. Exercise for abdominal and leg muscles   3 ×

12. Sirshasana (Rejuvenation)   3 ×

13. Meditation (Unity)   5 min

14. Savasana (Perfect relaxation)   5 min

OM

Week 17

1. Abdominal, middle, upper, and complete Yoga breathing (Rest) 7 × each

2. Jalandhara-Bandha (Retain breath for 7–30 sec with chin pressing against the chest) Will-power 3 ×

3. Ha-breathing (Lying: vigorously) Purity 3 ×

4. Ha-breathing (Standing: vigorously) Purity 3 ×

5. Yastikasana (Stick posture) Figure and beauty 3 ×

6. Natapadasana (Figure and beauty) 3 ×

7. Parshva-Pada-calanasana (Figure and beauty) 3 ×

8. Ardha-Matsyendrasana (Strong nerves) 2 ×

9. Trikonasana (Variation) Strong nerves 3 ×

10. Uddiyana-Bandha (Standing) Self-control 3 ×

11. Foot exercises 3 min

12. Halasana (Elasticity) 3 ×

13. Meditation (Unity) 5 min

14. Savasana (Perfect relaxation) 5 min

OM

Week 18

1. Abdominal, middle, upper, and complete Yoga breathing (Prana body development) 7 × each

2. Jalandhara-Bandha (Retain breath for 7–30 sec with chin pressing against the chest) Will-power 3 ×

3. Pranayama No. 4 (Strength) 3 ×

4. Agnisara Dhauti (Accelerated abdominal breathing) Purity 3 × 15 ×

5. Development of solar energy 3 min

6. Yoga-Mudra (Variation: to right and left) Health 3 ×

7. Lauliki-Yoga (Abdominal massage) 3 ×

8. Ardha-Matsyendrasana (Strong nerves) 3 ×

9. Kaakaasana (Raven posture) Security 3 ×

10. Mayurasana (Stability) 3 ×

11. Uddiyana-Bandha (Standing) Self-control 3 ×

12. Sirshasana or Sarvangasana (Rejuvenation) 3 ×

13. Meditation (Unity) 5 min

14. Savasana (Perfect relaxation) 5 min

OM

Week 19

1. Abdominal, middle, upper, and complete Yoga breathing (Prana body development) — 7 × each

2. Jalandhara-Bandha (Retain breath for 7–30 sec with chin pressing against the chest) Will-power — 3 ×

3. I.A.O.OM — 3 ×

4. Ardha-Ha-breathing (Lying) Purity — 3 ×

5. Pavanamuktasana (Clasp the knees tightly) Health — 3 ×

6. Vakrasana (Strong nerves) — 3 ×

7. Ardha-Matsyendrasana (Strong nerves) — 3 ×

8. Trikonasana (Variation) Strong nerves — 3 ×

9. Ardha-Chandrasana I (Elasticity) — 2 ×

10. Ardha-Chandrasana II (Elasticity) — 2 ×

11. Trataka (Fixation of point) — 3 min

12. Ardha-Sarvangasana (Rejuvenation) — 3 ×

13. Meditation (Unity) — 5 min

14. Savasana (Perfect relaxation) — 5 min

OM

Week 20

1. Abdominal, middle, upper, and complete
   Yoga breathing (Rest)   7 ×
   each

2. Jalandhara-Bandha (Retain breath for
   7–30 sec with chin pressing against the
   chest) Will-power   3 ×

3. Bhastrika (Bellows-breathing alternating)
   Purity   3 ×

4. Sitali (Inhale through tube-formed tongue)
   Blood cleansing   14 ×

5. Tadaghi-Mudra (Draw abdomen in tight)
   Resistance   3 ×

6. Stambhasana (Strength)   3 ×

7. Urdva-Paschimotanasana (Strength)   3 ×

8. Natashira-Vajrasana (Strength)   3 ×

9. Ekapadahastasana I (Figure and beauty)   2 ×

10. Ekapadahastasana II (Figure and beauty)   2 ×

11. Salabhasana (Kidneys) Purity   3 ×

12. Sirshasana or Sarvangasna (Rejuvenation)   3 ×

13. Meditation (Unity)   5 min

14. Savasana (Perfect relaxation)   5 min

OM

98

Week 21

1. Abdominal, middle, upper, and complete Yoga breathing (Rest) — 7 × each

2. Jalandhara-Bandha (Retain breath for 7–30 sec with chin pressing against the chest) Will-power — 3 ×

3. Bhastrika (Accelerated complete breathing) Purity — 3 × 7 ×

4. Development of solar energy — 3 min

5. Paschimotanasana (Health) — 3 ×

6. Pavanamuktasana (Lying: clasp the knees tightly) Health — 3 × 7 ×

7. Dolasana (Elasticity) — 3 ×

8. Kaakaasana (Raven posture) Equilibrium — 3 ×

9. Padangustasana (Equilibrium) — 3 ×

10. Chakrasana (Elasticity) — 3 ×

11. Hastapadangustasana (Strength) — 3 ×

12. Sirshasana or Sarvangasana (Rejuvenation) — 3 ×

13. Meditation (Unity) — 5 min

14. Savasana (Perfect relaxation) — 5 min

OM

Week 22

1. Abdominal, middle, upper, and complete Yoga breathing (Rest) — 7 × each

2. Jalandhara-Bandha (Retain breath for 7–30 sec with chin pressing against the chest) Will-power — 3 ×

3. Pranayama No. 1 (Self-control) — 3 ×

4. Pranayama No. 2 (Resistance) — 3 ×

5. Ardha-Matsyendrasana I (Self-confidence) — 2 ×

6. Ardha-Matsyendrasana II (Strong nerves) — 3 ×

7. Ekapadahastasana I (Figure and beauty) — 2 ×

8. Ekapadahastasana II (Figure and beauty) — 2 ×

9. Natarajasana (Equilibrium) — 3 ×

10. Simhasana (Tongue exercise) — 3 min

11. Eye-strengthening exercises (Bru-Madya-Drishti: fixation between the eyebrows. Nasagra-Drishti: fixation of nose tip) — 2 × each

12. Ardha-Halasana (Feet over right shoulder and then over left) Elasticity — 3 ×

13. Meditation (Unity) — 5 min

14. Savasana (Perfect relaxation) — 5 min

OM

Week 23

1. Abdominal, middle, upper, and complete Yoga breathing (Rest)   7 × each

2. Jalandhara-Bandha (Retain breath for 7-30 sec with chin pressing against the chest) Will-power   3 ×

3. Ha-breathing (Seated: inhale deeply, retain breath for 7 sec, exhale breath sharply and vigorously through the mouth) Purity   3 ×

4. Agnisara Dhauti (Accelerated abdominal breathing lying) Purity   2 × 14 ×

5. Kaakaasana (Raven posture) Strength   3 ×

6. Salabhasana (Kidneys) Purity   3 ×

7. Dhanurasana (Kidneys) Purity   3 ×

8. Stambhasana (Strength)   3 ×

9. Mayurasana (Strength)   3 ×

10. Ardha-Matsyendrasana (Strong nerves)   2 ×

11. Uddiyana-Bandha (Standing) Self-control   3 ×

12. Sirshasana or Sarvangasana (Rejuvenation)   3 ×

13. Meditation (Unity)   5 min

14. Savasana (Perfect relaxation)   5 min

OM

Week 24

1. Abdominal, middle, upper, and complete Yoga breathing (Rest)　　　7 × each

2. Jalandhara-Bandha (Retain breath for 7–30 sec with chin pressing against the chest) Will-power　　　3 ×

3. Sukh-purvak (Alternating breathing) Harmony and equilibrium　　　3 ×

4. I.A.O.OM　　　3 ×

5. Paschimotanasana (Health)　　　3 ×

6. Parvatasana (Mountain posture) Figure and beauty　　　3 ×

7. Ardha-Matsyendrasana (Strong nerves)　　　2 ×

8. Trikonasana (Strong nerves)　　　3 ×

9. Uddiyana-Bandha (Variation) Figure and beauty　　　3 ×

10. Uddiyana-Bandha (In squatting posture) Self-control　　　3 ×

11. Foot exercises　　　3 min

12. Halasana (Elasticity)　　　3 ×

13. Meditation (Unity)　　　5 min

14. Savasana (Perfect relaxation)　　　5 min

OM

Week 25

1. Abdominal, middle, upper, and complete   7 ×
   Yoga breathing (Prana body development)   each

2. Jalandhara-Bandha (Retain breath for
   7–30 sec with chin pressing against the
   chest) Will-power   3 ×

3. Sukh-purvak   (Alternating   breathing)
   Harmony   3 ×

4. I.A.O.O M   3 ×

5. Ustrasana (Elasticity)   3 ×

6. Yoga-Mudra (With fist on abdomen)   3 ×

7. Lauliki-Yoga (Abdominal massage)   3 ×

8. Uddiyana-Bandha (In squatting posture)
   Self-control   3 ×

9. Uddiyana-Bandha (Standing) Self-control   3 ×

10. Trikonasana (Variation) Strong nerves   3 ×

11. Supta-Vajrasana (Elasticity)   3 ×

12. Halasana (Resistance)   3 ×

13. Meditation (Unity)   5 min

14. Savasana (Perfect relaxation)   5 min

OM

Week 26

1. Abdominal, middle, upper, and complete Yoga breathing (Rest) — 7 × each

2. Jalandhara-Bandha (Retain breath for 7–30 sec with chin pressing against the chest) Will-power — 3 ×

3. Pranayama No. 6 — 3 ×

4. Pranayama No. 7 — 3 ×

5. Vibhakta-Janusirasana (Health) — 3 ×

6. Janusirasana (Horizontal) Strength — 2 ×

7. Janusirasana (Vertical) Strength — 2 ×

8. Vakrasana (Strong nerves) — 2 ×

9. Ardha-Chandrasana I (Elasticity) — 2 ×

10. Ardha-Chandrasana II (Elasticity) — 2 ×

11. Uddiyana-Bandha (Standing) Self-control — 3 ×

12. Halasana (Resistance) — 3 ×

13. Meditation (Unity) — 5 min

14. Savasana (Perfect relaxation) — 5 min

OM

Week 27

1. Abdominal, middle, upper, and complete Yoga breathing (Prana body development)   7 × each

2. Jalandhara-Bandha (Retain breath for 7–30 sec with chin pressing against the chest) Will-power   3 ×

3. Pranayama No. 6   3 ×

4. Pranayama No. 7   3 ×

5. Lauliki-Yoga (Health)   3 ×

6. Yoga-Mudra (With fist on abdomen) Health   3 ×

7. Ekapadahastasana I (Figure and beauty)   2 ×

8. Ekapadahastasana II (Figure and beauty)   2 ×

9. Natarajasana (Equilibrium)   3 ×

10. Vrksasana (Equilibrium)   3 ×

11. Development of solar energy   3 min

12. Viparita-Karani (Rejuvenation)   3 ×

13. Meditation (Unity)   5 min

14. Savasana (Perfect relaxation)   5 min

OM

Week 28

1. Abdominal, middle, upper, and complete Yoga breathing (Rest) — 7 × each

2. Jalandhara-Bandha (Retain for 7–30 sec with chin pressing against the chest) Will-power — 3 ×

3. Ha-breathing (Lying: vigorously) Purity — 3 ×

4. I.A.O.OM — 3 ×

5. Vakrasana (Strong nerves) — 2 ×

6. Ardha-Matsyendrasana (Strong nerves) — 2 ×

7. Trikonasana (Strong nerves) — 3 ×

8. Padahastasana (Strength) — 3 ×

9. Pavanamuktasana (Lying: clasp the knees tightly) Health — 3 × 9 ×

10. Bhegasana (Elasticity) — 3 ×

11. Vibhakta-Janusirasana (Resistance) — 3 ×

12. Viparita-Karani (Rejuvenation) — 3 ×

13. Meditation (Unity) — 5 min

14. Savasana (Perfect relaxation) — 5 min

OM

Week 29

1. Abdominal, middle, upper, and complete Yoga breathing (Rest) 7 × each

2. Breathe in deeply, exhale vigorously, squeeze out the air, tense the chest and abdominal muscles, retain breath for 7 sec, then quietly inhale and exhale deeply (Resistance) 3 ×

3. Agnisara Dhauti (Accelerated abdominal breathing, lying) Purity 2 × 9 ×

4. Development of solar energy 3 min

5. Padangustasana (Equilibrium) 3 ×

6. Natashira-Vajrasana (Strength) 3 ×

7. Matsyasana (Rest) 3 ×

8. Supta-Vajrasana (Elasticity) 3 ×

9. Trikonasana (Variation) Strong nerves 3 ×

10. Bhegasana (Elasticity) 3 ×

11. Natapadasana (Strength) 3 ×

12. Viparita-Karani (Rejuvenation) 3 ×

13. Meditation (Unity) 5 min

14. Savasana (Perfect relaxation) 5 min

OM

Week 30

1. Abdominal, middle, upper, and complete Yoga breathing (Prana body development)   7 × each

2. Jalandhara-Bandha (Retain breath for 7–30 sec with chin pressing against the chest) Will-power   3 ×

3. I.A.O.OM   3 ×

4. Mantrams:
My power of resistance is growing from moment to moment.
My will-power is growing from moment to moment.
Every organ is working better and better from moment to moment.
The cause of every bodily disorder is vanishing.
I manifest life in body and mind.
Rest and peace.
OM   3 × each

5. Padahastasana (Health)   3 ×

6. Hastapadangustasana (Strength)   3 ×

7. Natarajasana (Equilibrium)   3 ×

8. Matsyasana (Perfect relaxation)   3 ×

9. Salabhasana (Kidneys) Purity   3 ×

10. Dhanurasana (Kidneys) Purity   3 ×

11. Foot exercises   5 min

12. Sirshasana (Rejuvenation)   3 ×

13. Meditation (Unity)   5 min

14. Savasana (Perfect relaxation)   5 min

OM

Week 31

1. Abdominal, middle, upper, and complete Yoga breathing (Rest) — 7 × each

2. Jalandhara-Bandha (Retain breath for 7–30 sec with chin pressing against the chest) Will-power — 3 ×

3. Ha-breathing (Lying: vigorously) Purity — 3 ×

4. Ha-breathing (Standing: vigorously) Purity — 3 ×

5. Paschimotanasana (Health) — 3 ×

6. Yastikasana (Stick posture) Figure and beauty — 3 ×

7. Urdva-Paschimotanasana (Resistance) — 3 ×

8. Matsyasana (Regeneration of thyroid) — 3 ×

9. Supta-Vajrasana (Revitalising posture) — 3 ×

10. Bhegasana (Elasticity) — 3 ×

11. Ekapadahastasana I (Figure and beauty) — 3 ×

12. Ekapadahastasana II (Figure and beauty) — 3 ×

13. Sirshasana (Complete relaxation and rejuvenation) — 3 ×

14. Meditation (Unity) — 5 min

15. Savasana (Perfect relaxation) — 5 min

OM

Week 32

1. Abdominal, middle, upper, and complete Yoga breathing (Rest) 7 × each

2. Jalandhara-Bandha (7–30 sec with chin pressing against chest) Will-power 3 ×

3. Breathe in deeply and expel all breath, tense the chest and abdominal muscles and do not breathe for 7 sec. Inhale deeply 3 ×

4. Agnisara Dhauti (Accelerated abdominal breathing) Purity 15–30 × 3 ×

5. Kaakaasana (Raven posture) Equilibrium 3 ×

6. Dhrityasana (Resolution) 3 ×

7. Dhanurasana (Elasticity) 3 ×

8. Salabhasana (Kidneys) Purity 3 ×

9. Yoga-Mudra (Variation II with retention of breath) Resolution 3 ×

10. Padahastasana (Health) 3 ×

11. Sarvangasana (Variation) Rejuvenation 3 ×

12. Halasana (With legs apart) Elasticity 3 ×

13. Meditation (Unity) 5 min

14. Savasana (Perfect relaxation) 5 min

OM

Week 33

1. Abdominal, middle, upper, and complete Yoga breathing (Rest) — 7 × each

2. Jalandhara-Bandha (Retain breath for 7–30 sec with chin pressing against the chest) Will-power — 3 ×

3. Chest-tapping exercise (Breathe in slowly, rapidly tap the chest with the fingertips. Hold breath. Slap chest with palms of hands. Slowly exhale) Cleansing of lungs — 3 ×

4. Sukh-purvak (Alternating breathing) Harmony and equilibrium — 3 ×

5. Ardha-Chandrasana I (Elasticity) — 3 ×

6. Ardha-Chandrasana II (Elasticity) — 3 ×

7. Gomukhasana (Strength) — 3 ×

8. Urdva-Paschimotanasana (Resistance) — 3 ×

9. Chakrasana (Figure and beauty) — 3 ×

10. Trikonasana (Strong nerves) — 3 ×

11. Uddiyana-Bandha (Standing) Self-control — 3 ×

12. Ardha-Sarvangasana (Rest) — 3 ×

13. Ardha-Halasana (Elasticity) — 3 ×

14. Meditation (Unity) — 5 min

15. Savasana (Perfect relaxation) — 5 min

OM

Week 34

1. Abdominal, middle, upper, and complete Yoga breathing (Rest) — 7 × each

2. Jalandhara-Bandha (Retain breath for 7–21 sec with chin pressing into chest) Will-power — 3 ×

3. 'S' breathing (Purity) — 3 ×

4. Sukh-purvak (Alternating respiration) — 3 ×

5. Ardha-Bhujangasana I (Elasticity) — 3 ×

6. Ardha-Bhujangasana II (Elasticity) — 3 ×

7. Vakrasana (Variation: turn to right and left) — 3 ×

8. Sarpasana (Strength) — 3 ×

9. Hastapadangustasana (Stability) — 3 ×

10. Vrksasana (Equilibrium) — 3 ×

11. Uddiyana-Bandha (Seated) Figure and beauty — 3 ×

12. Uddiyana-Bandha (Standing) Figure and beauty — 3 ×

13. Viparita-Karani (With eye-strengthening exercises) Rejuvenation — 3 ×

14. Meditation (Unity) — 5 min

15. Savasana (Perfect relaxation) — 5 min

OM

Week 35

1. Abdominal, middle, upper, and complete Yoga breathing (Rest) — 7 × each

2. Jalandhara-Bandha (Retain breath for 7–14 sec with chin pressing against the chest) Will-power — 3 ×

3. Cleansing breathing — 3 ×

4. Pranayama No. 4 (Strength) — 3 ×

5. Ardha-Matsyendrasana I (Self-confidence) — 2 ×

6. Ardha-Matsyendrasana II (Strong nerves) — 3 ×

7. Paschimotanasana (Health) — 3 ×

8. Padahastasana (Resistance) — 3 ×

9. Uddiyana-Bandha (Standing) Figure and beauty — 3 ×

10. Eye exercises (Bru-Madya-Drishti: fixation between eyebrows. Nasagra-Drishti: fixation of tip of nose) — 3 ×

11. Simhasana (Exhale, protrude tongue, inhale, arch tongue upwards and press hard against palate) — 3 × 7 ×

12. Viparita-Karani (Rejuvenation) — 2 × 7 ×

13. Meditation (Unity) — 5 min

14. Savasana (Perfect relaxation) — 5 min

OM

Week 36

1. Abdominal, middle, upper, and complete
   Yoga breathing (Rest) — 7 ×
   each

2. Jalandhara-Bandha (Retain breath for
   7–30 sec with chin pressing against the
   chest) Will-power — 3 ×

3. Agnisara Dhauti (Accelerated abdominal
   breathing, lying) Purity — 2 × 14 ×

4. Sitali (Inhale through tube-formed tongue)
   Purification of blood — 14 ×

5. Pavanamuktasana (Lying: clasp the
   knees tightly) Health — 3 ×

6. Ardha-Matsyendrasana (Strong nerves) — 2 ×

7. Ustrasana (Figure and beauty) — 3 ×

8. Urdva-Paschimotanasana (Resistance) — 3 ×

9. Natashira-Vajrasana (Strength) — 3 ×

10. Yastikasana (Stick posture) Figure and
    beauty — 3 ×

11. Trikonasana (Strong nerves) — 3 ×

12. Ardha-Sarvangasana (Rejuvenation) — 3 ×

13. Meditation (Unity) — 5 min

14. Savasana (Perfect relaxation) — 5 min

OM

Week 37

1. Abdominal, middle, upper, and complete Yoga breathing (Rest) — 7 × each

2. Inhale deeply, exhale vigorously, squeeze out the remaining air, tense chest and abdominal muscles, do not breathe for 7–10 sec, then quietly inhale and exhale deeply (Resistance) — 3 ×

3. Bhastrika (Bellows-breathing) Purity — 2 × 9 ×

4. Development of solar energy — 3 ×

5. Tadaghi-Mudra (Draw in abdomen tightly) Health — 3 ×

6. Yoga-Mudra (With fist on abdomen) Health — 3 ×

7. Bhujangendrasana (Elasticity) — 3 ×

8. Trikonasana (Strong nerves) — 3 ×

9. Lauliki-Yoga (Health) — 3 ×

10. Padahastasana (Health) — 3 ×

11. Foot exercises — 3 min

12. Viparita-Karani (Rejuvenation) — 3 ×

13. Meditation (Unity) — 5 min

14. Savasana (Perfect relaxation) — 5 min

OM

Week 38

1. Abdominal, middle, upper, and complete   7 ×
   Yoga breathing (Rest)   each

2. Jalandhara-Bandha (Retain breath for
   7–30 sec with chin pressing against the
   chest) Will-power   3 ×

3. I.A.O.O M   3 ×

4. Pranayama No. 4 (Strength)   3 ×

5. Padahastasana (Health)   3 ×

6. Uddiyana-Bandha (Squatting posture:
   draw abdomen in tightly)   3 ×

7. Uddiyana-Bandha (Standing) Self-control   3 ×

8. Uddiyana-Bandha (Lying: draw in abdomen tightly after exhalation) Self-control   3 ×

9. Vakrasana (Strong nerves)   3 ×

10. Chakrasana (Elasticity)   3 ×

11. Foot exercises   3 min

12. Halasana (Elasticity)   3 ×

13. Meditation (Unity)   5 min

14. Savasana (Perfect relaxation)   5 min

OM

Week 39

1. Abdominal, middle, upper, and complete Yoga breathing (Rest) — 7 × each

2. Jalandhara-Bandha (Retain breath for 7–30 sec with chin pressing against the chest) Will-power — 3 ×

3. Ha-breathing (Lying: vigorously) Purity — 3 ×

4. Ha-breathing (Standing: vigorously) Purity — 3 ×

5. Vajroli-Mudra (Resistance) — 3 ×

6. Yoga-Mudra (With fist on abdomen) Health — 3 ×

7. Dhanurasana (Kidneys) Purity — 3 ×

8. Bhujangendrasana (Spine) Strength — 3 ×

9. Vibhatka-Janusirasana (Resistance) — 3 ×

10. Trikonasana (Strong nerves) — 3 ×

11. Trataka (Fixation of point) — 3 min

12. Sirshasana or Viparita-Karani (Rejuvenation) — 3 ×

13. Meditation (Unity) — 5 min

14. Savasana (Perfect relaxation) — 5 min

OM

Week 40

1. Abdominal, middle, upper, and complete Yoga breathing (Rest) — 7 × each

2. Jalandhara-Bandha (Retain breath for 7–30 sec with chin pressing against the chest) Will-power — 3 ×

3. Pranayama No. 2 (Strength) — 3 ×

4. Pranayama No. 4 (Strength) — 3 ×

5. Konasana (Figure and beauty) — 3 ×

6. Kaakaasana (Resistance) — 3 ×

7. Mayurasana (Resistance) — 3 ×

8. Uddiyana-Bandha (Standing) Self-control — 3 ×

9. Natarajasana (Equilibrium) — 3 ×

10. Padangustasana (Equilibrium) — 3 ×

11. Paschimotanasana (Health) — 3 ×

12. Viparita-Karani (With hands on knees) Rejuvenation — 3 ×

13. Meditation (Unity) — 5 min

14. Savasana (Perfect relaxation) — 5 min

OM

Week 41

1. Abdominal, middle, upper, and complete Yoga breathing (Rest) — 7 × each

2. Jalandhara-Bandha (Retain breath for 7–30 sec with chin pressing against the chest) Will-power — 3 ×

3. Ha-breathing (Lying: vigorously) Purity — 3 ×

4. Ha-breathing (Standing: vigorously) Purity — 3 ×

5. Tadaghi-Mudra (Draw in abdomen tight) Resistance — 3 ×

6. Natapadasana (Figure and beauty) — 3 ×

7. Parshva Pada-calanasana (Figure and beauty) — 3 ×

8. Matsyasana (Rest) — 3 ×

9. Vakrasana (Strong nerves) — 3 ×

10. Yoga-Mudra (Health) — 3 ×

11. Ardha-Chandrasana (Figure and beauty) — 3 ×

12. Ardha-Sarvangasana (Rejuvenation) — 3 ×

13. Meditation (Unity) — 5 min

14. Savasana (Perfect relaxation) — 5 min

OM

Week 42

1. Abdominal, middle, upper, and complete Yoga breathing (Rest) — 7 × each

2. Jalandhara-Bandha (Retain breath for 7–30 sec with chin pressing against the chest) Will-power — 3 ×

3. Pranayama No. 1 (Resistance) — 3 ×

4. Pranayama No. 2 (Resistance) — 3 ×

5. Vajroli-Mudra (Resistance) — 3 ×

6. Hastapadasana (Regeneration of the nervous system) — 3 ×

7. Janusirasana (Vertical) Security — 3 ×

8. Janusirasana (Horizontal) Security — 3 ×

9. Matsyasana (Regeneration of the thyroid) — 3 ×

10. Supta-Vajrasana (Charging of solar plexus) — 3 ×

11. Ardha-Matsyendrasana II (Strong nerves) — 3 ×

12. Sirshasana (Headstand) Rejuvenation — 3 ×

13. Meditation (Unity) — 5 min

14. Savasana (Perfect relaxation) — 5 min

OM

Week 43

1. Abdominal, middle, upper, and complete Yoga breathing (Prana body development) — 7 × each

2. Jalandhara-Bandha (Retain breath for 7–30 sec with chin pressing against the chest) Will-power — 3 ×

3. Pranayama No. 1 (Resistance) — 3 ×

4. Pranayama No. 2 (Resistance) — 3 ×

5. Paschimotanasana (Health) — 3 ×

6. Pavanamuktasana (Seated: clasp the knees tightly) Health — 3 × 7 ×

7. Urdva-Paschimotanasana (Resistance) — 3 ×

8. Bhegasana (Elasticity) — 3 ×

9. Padangustasana (Equilibrium) — 3 ×

10. Ustrasana (Elasticity) — 3 ×

11. Foot exercises — 3 min

12. Viparita-Karani (With tongue exercise) Simhasana (Rejuvenation) — 3 ×

13. Meditation (Unity) — 5 min

14. Savasana (Perfect relaxation) — 5 min

OM

Week 44

1. Abdominal, middle, upper, and complete Yoga breathing (Prana body development) — 7 × each

2. Jalandhara-Bandha (Retain breath for 7–30 sec with chin pressing against the chest) Will-power — 3 ×

3. Agnisara Dhauti (Accelerated abdominal respiration) Purity — 3 × 15 ×

4. Sitkari (Breathe in between tip of tongue and palate) Blood cleansing — 2 × 10 ×

5. Pavanamuktasana (Clasp the knees tightly) Health — 2 × 10 ×

6. Stambhasana (Strength) — 3 ×

7. Urdva-Paschimotanasana (Strength) — 3 ×

8. Natashira-Vajrasana (Strength) — 3 ×

9. Dhanurasana (Kidneys) Purity — 3 ×

10. Mayurasana (Resistance) — 3 ×

11. Vrksasana (Balance and Harmony) — 3 ×

12. Sarvangasana (Rejuvenation) — 3 ×

13. Meditation (Unity) — 5 min

14. Savasana (Perfect relaxation) — 5 min

OM

Week 45

1. Abdominal, middle, upper, and complete Yoga breathing (Rest) — 7 × each

2. Jalandhara-Bandha (Retain breath for 7–21 sec with chin pressing against the chest) Will-power — 3 ×

3. Sukh-purvak (4–16–8 sec) Harmony and equilibrium — 3 ×

4. Agnisara Dhauti (Accelerated abdominal breathing) Purity — 2 × 14 ×

5. Uddiyana-Bandha (In squatting posture) Self-control — 3 ×

6. Parshva Pada-calanasana (Strength) — 3 ×

7. Katikasana (Figure and beauty) — 3 ×

8. Uttha-Janusirasana (Resistance) — 3 ×

9. Natashira-Vajrasana (Strength) — 3 ×

10. Urdva-Paschimotanasana (Security) — 3 ×

11. Bhujangendrasana (Strong nerves) — 3 ×

12. Viparita-Karani (With eye-strengthening exercises) Rejuvenation — 3 ×

13. Meditation (Unity) — 5 min

14. Savasana (Perfect relaxation) — 5 min

OM

Week 46

1. Abdominal, middle, upper, and complete Yoga breathing (Rest) — 7 × each

2. Jalandhara-Bandha (Retain breath for 7–30 sec with chin pressing against the chest) Will-power — 3 ×

3. Cleansing breathing — 3 ×

4. Nerve-strengthening breathing — 3 ×

5. Lauliki-Yoga (Abdominal massage) — 3 ×

6. Yoga-Mudra (With fist on abdomen) Health — 3 ×

7. Bhujangendrasana (Spine) Strong nerves — 3 ×

8. Ardha-Salabhasana (Kidneys) Purity — 3 ×

9. Salabhasana (Kidneys) Purity — 3 ×

10. Padahastasana (Health) — 3 ×

11. Mantrams:
    My power of resistance is growing from moment to moment.
    Every organ is working better and better from moment to moment.
    The cause of every bodily disorder is vanishing.
    I manifest life in body and mind.
    Rest and peace.
    O M—O M—O M — 3 × each

12. Sarvangasana (Rejuvenation) — 3 ×

13. Meditation (Unity) — 5 min

14. Savasana (Perfect relaxation) — 5 min

OM

Week 47

1. Abdominal, middle, upper, and complete Yoga breathing (Prana body development) — 7 × each

2. Jalandhara-Bandha (Retain breath for 30 sec with chin pressing against the chest) Will-power — 3 ×

3. Chest-tapping exercise (Purity) — 3 ×

4. Bhastrika (Accelerated complete breathing) Purity — 2 × 7 ×

5. Vajroli-Mudra (Resistance) — 3 ×

6. Stambhasana (Strength) — 3 ×

7. Urdva-Paschimotanasana (Resistance) — 3 ×

8. Katikasana (Elasticity) — 3 ×

9. Bhujangasana (Kidneys) Purity — 3 ×

10. Dhanurasana (Kidneys) Purity — 3 ×

11. I.A.O.OM — 3 ×

12. Halasana (Elasticity) — 3 ×

13. Meditation (Unity) — 5 min

14. Savasana (Perfect relaxation) — 5 min

OM

Week 48

1. Abdominal, middle, upper, and complete Yoga breathing (Rest) — 7 × each

2. Jalandhara-Bandha (Retain breath for 7–21 sec with chin pressing against the chest) Will-power — 3 ×

3. Sukh-purvak (4–16–8 sec) Harmony and equilibrium — 3 ×

4. Agnisara Dhauti (Accelerated abdominal breathing) Purity — 2 × 14 ×

5. Uddiyana-Bandha (In squatting posture) Self-control — 3 ×

6. Parshva Pada-calanasana (Strength) — 3 ×

7. Katikasana (Figure and beauty) — 3 ×

8. Uttha-Janusirasana (Resistance) — 3 ×

9. Natashira-Vajrasana (Strength) — 3 ×

10. Urdva-Paschimotanasana (Will-power and resistance) — 3 ×

11. Bhujangendrasana (Strong nerves) — 3 ×

12. Viparita-Karani (With eye-strengthening exercises) Rejuvenation — 3 ×

13. Meditation (Unity) — 5 min

14. Savasana (Perfect relaxation) — 5 min

OM

Week 49

1. Abdominal, middle, upper, and complete
   Yoga breathing (Prana body development)   7 ×
                                                            each

2. Jalandhara-Bandha (Retain breath for
   7–30 sec with chin pressing against the
   chest) Will-power   3 ×

3. Agnisara Dhauti (Accelerated abdominal
   breathing lying) Purity   3 × 15 ×

4. Sitali (Breathe in through tube-formed
   tongue) Purification of the blood   2 × 15 ×

5. Lauliki-Yoga (Abdominal massage)   3 ×

6. Pavanamuktasana (Clasp the knees
   tightly) Health   3 × 7 ×

7. Uddiyana-Bandha (In squatting posture:
   Draw in abdomen tightly)   3 ×

8. Trikonasana (Strong nerves)   3 ×

9. Ardha-Matsyendrasana I I (Strong nerves)   3 ×

10. Ardha-Bhujangasana (Elasticity)   3 ×

11. Ardha-Salabhasana (Kidneys) Purity   3 ×

12. Ardha-Sarvangasana (Thyroid)
    Rejuvenation   3 ×

13. Meditation (Unity)   5 min

14. Savasana (Perfect relaxation)   5 min

OM

Week 50

1. Abdominal, middle, upper, and complete Yoga breathing (Rest) — 7 × each

2. Jalandhara-Bandha (Retain breath for 7–30 sec with chin pressing against the chest) Will-power — 3 ×

3. Cleansing breathing — 3 ×

4. Breathing to strengthen the nerves — 3 ×

5. Stambhasana (Resistance) — 3 ×

6. Urdva-Paschimotanasana (Will-power and resistance) — 3 ×

7. Yastikasana (Stick posture) Figure and beauty — 3 ×

8. Parvatasana (Mountain posture) Figure and beauty — 3 ×

9. Bhujangendrasana (Kidneys) Purity — 3 ×

10. Dhanurasana (Kidneys) Purity — 3 ×

11. Foot exercises — 3 min

12. Sirshasana or Viparita-Karani (Rejuvenation) — 3 ×

13. Meditation (Unity) — 5 min

14. Savasana (Perfect relaxation) — 5 min

OM

Week 51

1. Abdominal, middle, upper, and complete Yoga breathing (Rest) — 7 × each

2. Jalandhara-Bandha (Retain breath for 7–30 sec with chin pressing against the chest) Will-power — 3 ×

3. 'S' breathing — 3 ×

4. I.A.O.OM — 3 ×

5. Pavanamuktasana (Clasp the knees tightly) Health — 3 × 7 ×

6. Yastikasana (Stick posture) Figure and beauty — 3 ×

7. Padangustasana (Equilibrium) — 3 ×

8. Gokarnasana (Figure and beauty) — 3 ×

9. Natarajasana (Equilibrium) — 3 ×

10. Kaakaasana (Raven posture) Equilibrium — 3 ×

11. Paschimotanasana (Health) — 3 ×

12. Viparita-Karani (Rejuvenation) — 3 ×

13. Viparita-Karani II (Support knees with hands) Rejuvenation — 3 ×

14. Meditation (Unity) — 5 min

15. Savasana (Perfect relaxation) — 5 min

OM

Week 52

1. Abdominal, middle, upper, and complete Yoga breathing (Rest) — 7 × each

2. Jalandhara-Bandha (Retain breath for 7–30 sec with chin pressing against the chest) Will-power — 3 ×

3. Pranayama No. 3 (Resistance) — 3 ×

4. Pranayama No. 4 (Strength) — 3 ×

5. Yoga-Mudra (With fist on abdomen) Health — 3 ×

6. Bhujangendrasana (Strong nerves) — 3 ×

7. Ardha-Salabhasana (Kidneys) — 3 ×

8. Padahastasana (Health) — 3 ×

9. Uddiyana-Bandha (Standing) Self-control — 3 ×

10. Uddiyana-Bandha (In squatting posture) Self-control — 3 ×

11. Ardha-Matsyendrasana II (Strong nerves) — 3 ×

12. Sirshasana (Headstand) Rejuvenation — 3 ×

13. Meditation (Unity) — 5 min

14. Savasana (Perfect relaxation) — 5 min

OM

4 New Pranayama Breathing Exercises, Hatha Yoga Exercises and their Therapeutic Effect

PRANAYAMA BREATHING EXERCISES

1. *Abdominal, middle, upper, and complete Yoga breathing*

Abdominal breathing
Stand, sit, or lie. Direct consciousness to the region of the navel. With the exhalation draw in the abdominal wall. Then, through the nose *breathe in* slowly while relaxing the diaphragm; arch the abdominal wall outward, and fill up the lower part of the lungs with air. *Exhalation*: draw the abdominal wall in tightly, forcing the air out of the lungs through the nose. In abdominal breathing, only the lower lobes of the lungs are filled with air and thus only the abdomen executes a wavelike movement, while the *chest remains motionless*.

Therapeutic effect: A magnificent relaxation for the heart. Reduces high blood pressure, stimulates digestion, regulates intestinal activity. Abdominal breathing gives a splendid internal massage to all organs of the abdomen.

Middle breathing
Stand, sit, or lie. Direct the consciousness to the ribs. After exhaling, *inhale slowly* through the nose while expanding the ribs to both sides. In *exhaling*, contract the ribs, thus forcing the air out through the nose. In middle breathing the middle part of the lungs is filled with air, while *the abdomen and shoulders remain motionless*.

Therapeutic effect: Takes the pressure off the heart; freshens the blood circulation to the liver, gall-bladder, stomach, spleen, and kidneys.

Upper breathing

Stand, sit, or lie. Direct the consciousness to the top of the lungs. After exhaling, *breathe in* by slowly lifting the collar-bone and the shoulders, letting air flow in through the nose and fill the upper part of the lungs. In *exhaling*, slowly lower the shoulders and press the air out of the lungs through the nose. In upper breathing the *abdomen and the middle part of the chest remain motionless*.

Therapeutic effect: Strengthens the hilar lymph nodes in the lungs: thoroughly airs the tips of the lungs.

Complete Yoga breathing

Stand, sit, or lie. Animate the entire trunk by means of the consciousness, always following the wavelike movement of the inhalation and exhalation. Complete equilibrium is experienced. After exhaling, slowly breathe in through the nose, counting up to eight, and combining lower, middle and upper breathing in a wavelike movement (Puraka). First expand the abdomen, then the ribs, and finally raise the collar-bone. At this point, when the abdominal wall is already drawing in slightly, begin the exhalation (Rechaka) in the same manner as the inhalation, that is, by first drawing in the abdominal wall, then contracting the ribs and finally lowering the shoulders, while letting the air out through the nose. In complete Yoga breathing, the entire breathing mechanism, i.e. the lower, middle and upper lobes of the lungs, are in uniform movement. Between the inhalation and the exhalation the breath can be retained for as long as is comfortable.

Therapeutic effect: Completely airs the lungs, increases the oxygen and prana supply in the blood, sets up an equilibrium between the positive and negative currents, calms the entire nervous system, regulates and slows the activity of the heart, reduces high blood pressure, and stimulates digestion. Induces a feeling of peace, quiet, and security.

2. *Agnisara Dhauti*

Sit on the heels or lie flat on the back. With palms on the abdomen, exhale completely, slightly pressing the contracted region. With a short and abrupt breath, protrude the abdomen a little, immediately following with a quick expiration, simultaneously contracting the muscles of the abdomen like bellows. This should be done twenty to thirty times in quick succession. Never inhale completely, only take short breaths.   3 ×

Therapeutic effect: Purifies the blood and likewise each and every organ of the abdominal region. Eliminates constipation and its mental cause. Excellent for cleansing the skin and against liver disorders. Cures diabetes.

3. Ardha-Ha-breathing

Lie flat on the back. Inhale slowly with the complete Yoga breathing raising the arms above the head. Suddenly exhaling through the mouth, clasp the right knee with both hands. After 10 sec, inhale slowly lowering the right leg to the ground, raising the arms above the head. Suddenly exhaling through the mouth, clasp the left knee. Breathing in, raise the arms and, exhaling slowly through the nose, bring the arms down to the side.   3 ×

Therapeutic effect: Cleansing of the abdominal organs, right and left side alternately. Highly beneficial for disorders of the circulation.

4. Pranayama against Shortness of Breath

Inhale deeply as in full Yoga breathing. Exhale completely, dispelling the air from the lungs as much as possible. Contract the chest, the ribs and the abdomen. After 10–15 sec inhale again deeply.

5. Bhastrika (Bellows)

This exercise is the complete Yoga breathing with the only difference that it is performed with an accelerated rhythm.

Sit with your legs crossed or sit on the heels and exhale. Fill the lungs suddenly in the sequence abdominal, middle and upper breathing. Without a pause suddenly exhale, emptying the lungs by first contracting the abdominal wall, then the ribs and finally relaxing the shoulders. Do this 7–10 times consecutively.

2 ×

Therapeutic effect: Each time we inhale, the body cleanses itself with blood saturated with oxygen. The toxins are naturally discarded from the body:

(*a*) When breathing out.
(*b*) Through all the pores of the skin.
(*c*) In the form of perspiration.
(*d*) Through urine.
(*e*) Through excrement.

The elimination of toxins is greatly enhanced through the bellows movement of the lungs.

6. *Breathing to strengthen the nerves**

Stand with feet apart and, after exhaling, inhale slowly and at the same time raise both arms in front, palms upwards, until level with the shoulders. Then double the fists, and while still holding the breath, draw them back quickly to the shoulders, extend the arms, draw them back again quickly, and repeat this movement once more. While exhaling, relax the arms, letting them sink and rest while bending forward.

Therapeutic effect: Increases the resistance of the nervous system.

7. *Chest-tapping Exercise*

Sit with crossed legs. While inhaling very slowly, quickly tap the chest with the fingertips. Breath retention for about 7 sec, during which time pat the chest all over with the palms. Exhale. Repeat after a rest.

3 ×

Therapeutic effect: Excellent for pulmonary and bronchial catarrh, even for its variant form, bronchial asthma. As with all Yoga exercises the cause of the disease is removed.

8. *Cleansing Breathing**

Stand with legs apart and inhale slowly through the nose as in complete Yoga breathing. When the lungs are completely filled with air, exhale as follows: press the lips close to the teeth while keeping a narrow slit open between them. Through this narrow slit force the air out in a number of short, detached movements, using the abdominal, diaphragmatic and rib muscles vigorously to overcome the resistance.

Therapeutic effect: Expels the toxins in the blood and fortifies immunity.

9. *Ha-breathing (Lying)**

Lie flat on the back and inhale, as in full Yoga breathing, simultaneously raising the arms slowly until they reach the floor behind the head. Retain the breath for a few seconds and then quickly raise the legs, suddenly flex the knees, and, putting the arms about them, press the thighs to the abdomen and simultaneously breathe out with 'ha' breathing. The 'H A' sound is made by the rush of air itself and not the throat. After a few seconds rest, breathe in again slowly, raising the arms over the head, and at the same time stretching the legs upward and slowly lowering them to the floor. After a few seconds pause, slowly exhale through the nose while lowering the arms to the side of the trunk.

Therapeutic effect: Purges mental poisons and quickly dispels feelings of depression. Regenerates the inner organs.

10. *Ha-breathing (Standing)**

Stand with feet apart and inhale as in complete Yoga breathing. Inhale and raise the arms slowly vertically over the head, hold the breath for a few seconds, then, suddenly bending forward, let the arms drop down in front while simultaneously exhaling through the mouth and pronouncing the sound 'ha'. Then inhale slowly, straightening up, and again raising the arms vertically over the head. Then exhale slowly through the nose while lowering the arms.

Therapeutic effect: Similar to that of 'ha' breathing lying.

11. *I.A.O.0 M*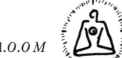

Just as a light ray passing through a glass prism resolves into seven colours, in the same way does the sound 'OM' contain all the existing sounds. Every Yogi experiences the same truth in his enlightenment, that sound is the first manifestation of God, and with IT creation begins. 'In the beginning was Logos, and Logos was with God and Logos was God,' says the Bible. Everything in this universe is created and animated by the creative force called LOGOS. Sound is the creative vibration which penetrates the universe and creates worlds. When we repeat certain sounds, we produce a curative effect in the body and simultaneously raise our consciousness to a higher level. The vibration of the sound IIIIII ... (pronounced as in marine) penetrates the whole nervous system, charging it with new vital force.

The repetition of the sound AAAAAA ... (as in after) has a special effect on the liver, and through it regenerates the blood. The repetition of the sound OOOOOO ... (as in over) charges the organ of the heart and the great nervous centre, the solar plexus, with vital force. The repetition of the sound OM charges the whole organism with new vital force.

Sit with legs crossed or sit on the heels with hands on the knees and the eyes closed. Inhale deeply and when exhaling repeat

the sound IIIIIII . . . prolonging the sound at the same pitch. *The sound must not be sung but spoken.*
Inhale deeply and when exhaling repeat the sound AAAAAA . . . in a prolonged manner and without raising or dropping the voice.
When exhaling for the third time repeat the sound OOOOOO . . . and finally the sound OOOOMMMM. . . .

Therapeutic effect: The voice becomes crystal-clear and pleasant to listen to, firm and self-confident. States of anxiety disappear and there is a conscious manifestation of the human spirit.

12. *Jalandhara-Bandha*

Sit with crossed legs. Inhale deeply. Retain the breath (from 7–30 sec) with the chin pressing against the chest. Then raise the head and slowly exhale.   3 ×

Therapeutic effect: Helps to raise the power of resistance and the will-power.

13. *Pranayama Exercises* (Nos 1–7)*

No. 1: Stand with the feet apart and raise the arms while slowly breathing in until the palms of the hands touch each other above the head. Hold the breath for 7–12 sec and then slowly lower the arms, palms down, while exhaling. Conclude the exercise with cleansing breathing.

No. 2: Stand with feet apart and inhale as in full Yoga breathing, arms forward, level with shoulders, palms of the hands downwards. While retaining the breath swing the arms rapidly and rhythmically back and outward as far as possible horizontally, then forward and backward again from three to five times; exhale vigorously through the mouth while slowly lowering the arms; conclude the exercise with cleansing breathing.

No. 3: Stand with feet apart. During slow inhaling as in full Yoga breathing, raise the arms forward to shoulder height with palms in. While retaining the breath, briskly swing the arms like a windmill upward, backward and around again, three times; then do the same in the opposite direction. Exhale vigorously through the mouth while the arms are lowered. Conclude with cleansing breathing.

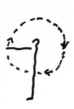

No. 4: Lie on the floor, face down, and put the palms of the hands on the floor under the shoulders, fingers forward. After a full inhalation retain the breath and do a slow push-up, holding the body stiff so that it rests only on the toes and hands. Slowly we lower the body to the floor again and repeat the movement three to five times. Exhale vigorously through the mouth. Conclude the exercise with cleansing breathing.

No. 5: Stand erect facing a wall, and put the palms of the hands on the wall at shoulder height, arms outstretched. After a full Yoga inhalation, retain the breath and lean forward, holding the body stiff, and bend the elbows until the forehead touches the wall; then by exerting our full strength, we push our body whilst holding it still, until it is vertical and erect again. Repeat three to five times, then exhale vigorously through the mouth. Conclude with cleansing breathing.

No. 6: Stand upright, straight as an arrow, feet apart, and hands on hips. After a full Yoga inhalation, hold the breath briefly, then bend forward slowly, breathing out through the nose as we bend. While slowly breathing in, straighten up again; then after a short retention of breath, breathe out while bending backwards. While breathing in again, straighten up; then do the same while bending to the right and straightening up again. While breathing out, bend to the left, then

138

straighten up while breathing in. After a short
retention of breath, breathe out calmly through
the nose while lowering the arms. Conclude with
cleansing breathing.

N. 7: Stand erect with feet apart or sit in the
Padmasana posture. Make a full Yoga inhalation,
but instead of drawing in the air in one movement,
inhale in short, detached puffs until the lungs are
completely full. Retain the breath 7–12 sec, then
then breathe out through the nose calmly and
slowly. Conclude with cleansing breathing.

14. 'S' Breathing

Sit with legs crossed. Inhale deeply. When exhaling repeat the
sound 'S' (as in hi*ss*) prolonging it. Let it be very clear.   3 ×

Therapeutic effect: Strengthens the nerves and raises the powers
of resistance.

15. Sitali

Sit with legs crossed. Forming a tube with the tongue, protrude
it a little out of the mouth. Inhale slowly through the tube-
formed tongue. Retain the breath (for up to 10 sec), then
exhale slowly and relaxed through the nose. Repeat ten times
consecutively.   3 ×

Therapeutic effect: Immediate relaxation of the nerves. Very
effective against breathing difficulties, heart troubles and
extreme nervousness. Removes all toxins from the blood, even
deadly poisons. Regenerates the skin and gives a beautiful
complexion. In winter practise indoors only.

16. Sitkari

Sit with legs crossed. Differs from Sitali only in that the tip of
the tongue touches the back of the palate. Inhale very slowly
through the mouth letting the air pass between the tip of the
tongue and the palate. Retain the breath for 10 sec, then exhale

very slowly and completely relaxed through the nose. Perform about seven times in succession.   3 ×

Therapeutic effect: The same as with the previous exercise. Accelerates the elimination of toxins (poisonous matter) from the whole body.

17. *Sukh-purvak** (Comfortable Pranayama)

In Padmasana (Lotus Seat) place the right index finger on the centre of the forehead between the eyebrows. After a vigorous exhalation hold the right nostril closed with the right thumb, inhaling through the left nostril during four pulse beats. Retain the breath for sixteen beats, release the right nostril, place the middle finger on the left nostril and exhale through the right nostril during eight beats. Keep the fingers as they are. After inhaling through the right nostril during four beats and retaining the breath sixteen beats, close the right nostril and exhale through left during eight beats.

Therapeutic effect: Enhances mental functions and alertness.

18. *Development of Solar Energy*

The human body radiates vital energy which protects it and keeps it immune. This radiation of energy can be measured with a precision instrument such as may be used in an Atomic Research Institute. If this protective wall of energy is weakened, the body is at the mercy of external influences. If immunity is lost, the body gets ill. If the solar plexus has enough energy, the body is able to resist all external influences.

Execution: Lie flat on the back. Place the palms of the hands on the chest a little above the navel with fingers apart from each other. Inhale deeply filling the lungs with vital force. Exhale very slowly leading vital force from the lungs through the arms and fingers into the chest, into the solar plexus, the nerve centres of which are located at the spinal cord. Repeat fifteen to twenty times.

Therapeutic effect: Extremely effective against fatigue, insomnia and circulatory disorders.

HATHA YOGA EXERCISES

1. *Abdominal and leg-muscle exercises*

(*a*) The following exercises are excellent for the strengthening of the too often neglected abdominal region, the pelvis, the small of the back and the hips:

Lie flat on the back and inhale deeply. While exhaling sit up and raise the stretched right leg vertically, holding the ankles with both hands, to touch the knee with the forehead. Inhale and lie back again, exhaling, sit up and raise the left leg vertically to touch the knee with the forehead. Inhaling, lie back and rest. 3 ×

(*b*) Sit with the legs wide apart, hands on the ground behind the back. While inhaling, raise the waist as high above the ground as possible, but *very slowly and carefully*. Then exhaling, return slowly to the ground and lie flat on the back. Rest with deep abdominal breathing. 3 ×

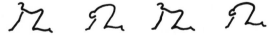

(*c*) Kneel with the hands on the ground. Without moving the body forward or backward, inhale, dipping the waist until the small of the back is hollow and at the same time raise the head. While exhaling, raise the waist, drawing in the abdomen and dropping the head. Repeat consecutively four to five times. Sitting on the heels, lean forward and support the head on the fists, placed one over the other. 3 ×

(*d*) Kneel again with hands on the ground. While inhaling, raise the right leg backward and raise the head. Exhale drawing the right knee up to the forehead. Inhale while raising the right leg backward, exhale bringing the right leg to the ground again. Repeat the same movement with the left leg. Repeat the exercise and return to the original kneeling position. 3 ×

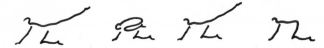

(*e*) Excellent for all the joints. Very good for flabby hips and for reducing fatty deposits on the abdomen. Kneel with hands on the ground. Inhale deeply. While exhaling, pass the right leg between the hands until it is stretched in front. Touch the right knee with the forehead and inhaling, draw back the right leg to its former position. Exhaling, slide the left leg forward bringing the forehead to touch the left knee. Inhale returning the left leg to the original position and exhaling, bend forward and rest.

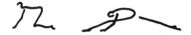

(*f*) Stand upright with legs wide apart from each other. While exhaling, bend forward and touch the ground with the palms, elbows and forehead. Remain breathing in this position for 5–10 sec. Stand up again with feet together. 3 ×

(*g*) This exercise is very effective for strengthening the spinal column, for disorders of the small of the back and low backache. Stand upright with feet together. Inhale, raising arms above the head. Exhale bending forward until the upper body is parallel to the ground. In this phase the posterior will move slightly backwards. Inhale straightening up, exhale bending forward again. Repeat in all three to five times consecutively, then rest.

2. Ardha-Bhujangasana*

Kneel on the left knee, putting the right forward so that the shin is vertical. Make a full Yoga inhalation. While exhaling, shift the weight from the left knee to the right foot and slowly lower the trunk until the hands, hanging downwards, touch the floor. Hold the backbone upright. Remain thus for 3–7 sec without breathing and then slowly rise during a full Yoga inhalation. Repeat three times and then change the feet.

Therapeutic effect: The resilience and elasticity of the entire bone structure are preserved and improved.

3. Ardha-Chandrasana I

Stand upright with feet together. Raise the chest and draw the abdomen in. Inhale deeply, raising the arms above the head, placing the palms together. Exhale while bending to the right side. Inhale while returning to the upright position. Exhale while bending over to the left side. Inhale returning to the upright position. Exhale—lower the arms from front. Repeat after a rest.   3 ×

Therapeutic effect: Improves our elasticity and prevents fatty deposits about the spine. Excellent against stiffness.

4. Ardha-Chandrasana II

Stand with feet apart. Inhaling, raise the arms above the head with palms together. Exhaling, bend back as far as possible with the knees slightly bent. Inhaling, return to the upright position. Exhaling, lower the arms from front.   3 ×

Therapeutic effect: The same as that of the previous exercise, only more powerful. The brisk circulation in chest, face and brain is excellent against fatigue.

143

5. *Ardha-Halasana*

Lie flat on the back, completely relaxed and take a deep breath. While exhaling raise the legs and the hips up and dip the feet to touch the ground at a wide angle from the right shoulder. Inhaling, stretch out legs and feet on the ground above the head. Exhaling, carry the legs over to the left shoulder. Keep this up, once to the right, once to the left, again to the right and again to the left. Then lower the legs and lie flat on the back. With deep abdominal breathing the heart works normally. 3 ×

Therapeutic effect: Strongly stimulates the activity of the thyroid glands. For those with sluggish digestion the grinding movement of the abdomen will stimulate the entire inner organism, particularly the peristaltic movement of the bowels. This exercise is highly recommended as a cure for constipation.

6. *Ardha-Matsyendrasana I**

Place the right heel under the left thigh with the right leg resting horizontally on the floor. Now put the left foot over the right thigh, setting the sole of the foot on the floor. Turn the chest to the left and put the right arm in front of the left knee which is vertically erect, and grasp the left ankle with the right hand. Slowly twist the back to the left, turning the head in the same direction. With the left arm reach backward and with the left hand grasp the left knee. Breathe with an even rhythm for as long as comfortable.

Therapeutic effect: Overcomes spinal deformities and benefits the entire nervous system.

7. Ardha-Matsyendrasana II*

This is an easier modification of the preceding exercise. Hold the spine upright without any twist and use complete Yoga breathing. Hold consciousness in the spine.

Therapeutic effect: Self-confidence, determination, and perseverance. Strengthens the nerves.

8. Ardha-Salabhasana*

The execution is the same as for Salabhasana except that one leg is raised and then the other, instead of both together.

Therapeutic effect: The same as that of Salabhasana, but less intense. This exercise requires much less exertion.

9. Ardha-Sarvangasana

Lie flat on the back and relax the body completely. Inhale deeply and while exhaling raise the legs and the hips up vertically. Still exhaling, bring the knees to touch the forehead while the legs are tucked in. Support the hips with the hands; regular, short abdominal breathing. After about 30 sec return legs to vertical position and lie flat on the back again. 3 ×

Therapeutic effect: The concentration of blood in the face and brain completely dispels fatigue. This exercise is indispensable for headaches caused by low blood-pressure and for giddy sensations in the brain as a result of poor circulation. The empty nerve cells of the brain are recharged with vital force.

145

10. *Bhegasana*

An exercise particularly designed for control of
the joints and for increasing elasticity. Lie flat on
the ground, bend the knees and grasp the toes of
both feet. Frequently press the feet to the ground
next to the hips. Repeat six times then let go of
the feet. Stretch out the legs and place the
hands under the forehead in order to rest.
Meanwhile breathe slowly.   3 ×

11. *Bhujangasana**

Lying face down on the floor, place both hands, palms down,
on the floor below the shoulders. With a full Yoga inhalation,
slowly raise the head as far as possible. Then tense the muscles
of the back and lift the shoulders and trunk higher and higher
and farther backwards without help from the arms. Remain in
this position and hold the breath for 7–12 sec, then breathe out
slowly and return to the prone position.

Therapeutic effect: Regenerates the entire abdomen and the
trunk.

12. *Bhujangendrasana*

An excellent massage for the ganglia, kidneys, neck and spinal
column. Vigorous circulation of blood in the spine removes
fatigue completely. Lie flat on the abdomen with hands below
the shoulders. Inhale raising the chest as high as possible,
simultaneously bending the knees so that the feet touch the
head from behind. Shortly afterwards exhale, lower the body
and lie flat on the abdomen to rest.   3 ×

13. *Bru-Madya-Drishti* (and Nasagra-Drishti)*

Sit in the Padmasana posture and inhale deeply, then breathe regularly and look at a spot between the eyebrows, i.e. a spot above the bridge of the nose. Pause at the slightest fatigue and practise Nasagra-Drishti. In this exercise look at the tip of the nose and remain in this posture breathing regularly until fatigued. See also 'Eye Exercises' and Trataka.

14. *Chakrasana*

This exercise gives us a complete control over the spine. The positive and negative vital currents, the solar and lunar energy known as HA-THA, are balanced. Clears blocked nostrils.

Lie flat on the back. Draw in the knees and place feet wide apart on the ground. Place hands backwards on the ground below the shoulders. Inhaling deeply, raise the whole body to form a bridge. While in this position breathe slowly and deeply. After a few seconds lower the body, lie flat on the back and relax completely.   3 ×

15. *Dhanurasana**

Lying on the floor, face down, inhale slowly, reach back, and grasp both ankles, arching the back and remaining in this posture as long as possible. During this exercise breathe slowly and hold the consciousness in the pelvic region.

Therapeutic effect: Stimulates the endocrine glands, especially the sexual glands. Postpones the symptoms of sexual weakness characteristic of the climacteric and preserves youth into old age.

16. *Dhrityasana*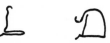

This exercise strengthens the pelvis, small of the back and abdomen. Removes fatigue in the small of the back.

Sit on the ground between the heels with knees apart. Hold

the ankles or heels with both hands. Inhaling deeply, raise the pelvis, small of the back and chest as high as possible, dropping back the head. Remain in this position for a few moments breathing deeply. Exhaling, place the knees and feet together and sitting on the heels, bend forward to rest the forehead on the fists placed one over the other. 3 ×

17. *Dolasana*

This exercise is recommended for the vitalising of the whole body as well as the consciousness and for the development of form and beauty. Lie on the abdomen with arms stretched out in front of you. Inhaling deeply, raise the arms, chest and legs as high as possible. While exhaling lower the body slowly with stretched arms. 3 ×

18. *Ekapadahastasana I*

Squat with palms of the hands on the ground, straighten the legs. While inhaling raise right leg, while exhaling bring leg down. Inhaling, raise left leg, exhaling, bring leg down. Repeat the same movement twice more. Sitting on the heels bend forward and rest. 3 ×

19. *Ekapadahastasana II*

Squat with palms of the hands on the ground, straighten the legs. While inhaling, raise right leg to the right side, while exhaling bring right leg down again. Perform the same with the left leg to the left side. (Be careful not to raise the leg to the rear, but to the side only.) Repeat again with each leg. Rest sitting on the heels.   3 ×

Therapeutic effect: Hips, abdomen, pelvis and legs are strongly exerted.

20. *Eye Exercises* (See also Bru-Madya-Drishti)*

Eye swinging: Look straight ahead. Inhale deeply and turn the eyes as far to the right as possible. Exhale slowly and return the eyes to looking straight ahead. Inhale again and turn the eyes to the left and then, on exhaling, back to the centre.

Eye rolling: Look straight ahead and then, while exhaling, look downward. While slowly inhaling, start to describe a circle with the eyes to the right and upward until they reach top centre. Then begin to exhale and continue to roll towards the left and downward until they reach bottom centre again. Begin again with inhalation and continue to the right and upwards until the circle has been completed three times. After a rest, roll the eyes in the other direction.

21. *Exercises for the feet*

Those who do this intensive Hatha Yoga training should practise the foot exercises daily for a few mins at any time of day. Walk round your room on the tips of the toes only for about 1 min. Then walk normally, that is, placing first heel, then sole, then toes to the ground.
After 1 min walk on the heels only with stiff knees and raising the toes. After 1 min walk normally again. Now walk on the side of the feet with stiff knees. After twenty to thirty steps walk normally again. Now walk with arched feet, that is to say, touching the ground only with the heel and big toe, and with stiff knees. The feet are so strongly arched that a ball the size of a shilling piece could be rolled under the arched foot.

Therapeutic effect: These exercises correct flat feet. They should, however, be practised daily.

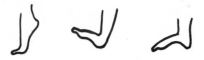

22. *Gokarnasana*

Makes the body conscious and helps achieve form and beauty. Lie on your back. Stretch the left arm above the head on the ground. Hold the right foot with the right hand and stretch it to the right side on the ground, so that both legs form a right angle. Remain in this position for about 20 sec with regular deep breathing. Repeat to the other side. 3 ×

23. *Gomukhasana*

This exercise strengthens the muscles of the shoulders, arms and back, and makes the joints of the upper body supple. Very effective against rheumatic pains as the circulation is stimulated in the joints.
Sitting on the heels, raise the left hand from below to the middle of the back, hold the left hand with the right hand from above so that the right elbow is pressed upwards. Perform alternately with the left and the right arm.

24. *Halasana**

Lie on the back with outstretched arms and hands, palms down, beside the thighs. Exhale slowly and lift both feet, carrying them beyond the head until the toes touch the floor. Keep the hands flat on the floor. Remain in this posture for 10–15 sec breathing slowly and regularly. This is the first phase. In the second phase push the feet much farther backwards, breathing deeply and ensuring that the knees are kept stiff. The weight is much more at the top of the spine. In the third phase the weight is supported by the vertebrae of the neck. Push the feet still farther back (knees still stiff), draw in the arms and clasp both hands behind the neck. Slowly unroll until the feet return to the starting position.

Therapeutic effect: Banishes fatigue or exhaustion. Makes the spine more supple.

25. *Halasana* (Variation)

Lying on the back raise legs and hips until the feet dip to the ground over the head. Remain in this position with legs apart for 15–20 sec with very relaxed breathing, then come down and lie completely relaxed.   3 ×

Therapeutic effect: Excellent for strengthening the spine and the small of the back.

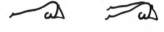

26. *Hastapadangustasana*

Stand upright. Raise the right knee and hold the ankle with both hands. Stretch out the leg to its full length for 7 to 10 sec, breathing slowly and deeply all the time. Then repeat with the left leg.   3 ×

Therapeutic effect: Gives self-confidence and self-reliance.

27. *Hastapadasana*

Sit with the legs wide apart. Inhale deeply, while exhaling bend forward holding the ankles, and if possible bring the

forehead to touch the ground. After about 5 sec sit up with
deep relaxed breathing. 3 ×

Therapeutic effect: An exceptionally effective exercise for spine,
small of the back, pelvis and legs.

28. *Janusirasana* (Vertical)

This exercise achieves perfect balance of the solar and lunar
energy, the positive and negative vital force in the whole body.
By increasing our power of resistance we develop a natural
immunity in the body. Sit with the right leg flexed and the left
leg raised vertically. Hold the left ankle with both hands and
touch the left knee with the forehead. Breathe in a very relaxed
manner. Repeat with the right leg. 3 ×

29. *Janusirasana* (Horizontal)

Sit with the right leg stretched out and the left
leg flexed so that the sole of the left foot touches
the inside of the right thigh. Bend over the right
leg and hold the foot or ankle with both hands.
At the same time turn the right shoulder downwards and the left shoulder upwards. Breathe
more slowly and deeply. Repeat with the left
leg. 3 ×

Therapeutic effect: Similar to that of the previous exercise.

30. *Kaakaasana* (Raven posture)

This exercise promotes a sense of balance and confidence as
well as resolution.
Squat on the toes with legs apart. Place hands on the ground

before you. Support the knees on the elbows and transfer the weight of the body to the upper arms and elbows. Try to draw up the feet—this can be achieved after some practice.

31. *Katikasana*

Sit on the ground, legs stretched and feet together, with the hands behind the body on the ground. While inhaling raise the pelvis as high as possible, and while exhaling return to sitting position. Repeat consecutively three or four times, then draw the knees together and rest with hands and forehead on the knees. 3 ×

Therapeutic effect: Of prime importance in vitalising the spine.

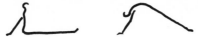

32. *Konasana*

Stand upright with legs apart, hands clasped behind the body. Inhale deeply, while exhaling bend over the right knee and, if possible, touch the knee with the forehead. Inhaling, stand upright, exhaling bend over the left knee. Inhaling, stand upright and exhaling remain upright. Deep and relaxed breathing. 3 ×

Therapeutic effect: Strengthens the inner organs and clears a sluggish stomach, liver and particularly intestines.

33. *Lauliki-Yoga*

Sit on the heels placing the hands on the abdomen. Inhaling

deeply, protrude the abdomen. While exhaling strongly press the whole abdominal wall from left to right with the hands. Inhaling, protrude the abdomen again, while exhaling again press it strongly from left to right. Perform another seven to ten times, then bend forward and rest.

3 ×

Therapeutic effect: Provides one of the best massages for all the organs of the abdominal cavity. Recommended for excess acidity, disorders of the pancreas, diabetes and constipation. To be avoided during menstruation.

34. *Maha-Mudra*

Sit with the right leg stretched and the left leg flexed, so that the left foot touches the inside of the right thigh. Bend over the right leg and hold the foot with both hands. Inhale deeply, exhaling strongly draw in the abdomen well, press the chest with the chin and at the same time close the anal muscle. Drawing in the abdomen = Uddiyana-Bandha; pressing the chin = Jalandhara-Bandha; closing the anal muscle = Mula-Bandha. After 5–7 sec inhale again and exhale. Perform the same to the left side.

Therapeutic effect: Enhances our will-power and powers of concentration and increases our resolution.

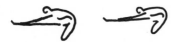

35. *Mantrams*

The development of energy through sounds is called Mantra-Yoga. This form of Yoga is also practised in India for physical health, for developing our power of concentration and for awaking the latent spiritual centres. The impressions of the day which result from thoughts, conversations, actions and deeds are stored in the subconscious mind. The practitioner of Yoga tries to gather positive, good, constructive impressions.
Sit up straight, eyes closed, shut out all thoughts and feelings.

Concentrating on the *I* in the heart centre, repeat the following thoughts softly or half-aloud:

I am free of all bonds. I am free. I am free.
My power of resistance is growing from moment to moment.
My will-power is growing from moment to moment.
The cause of every bodily disorder is vanishing.
                (Use only when necessary)
I am fearless. I am fearless. I am fearless.
I manifest life in mind and in body.
Perfect balance in mind and body.
Peace and rest. Peace and rest. Peace and rest.
I am conscious in mind and body.
Perfect health and strength.

Just as we water a plant at the root, so these commands invigorate, vitalise and liberate in all respects. These sentences may be spoken during the exercises or in bed, just before falling asleep. Practise daily.

36. *Matsyasana**

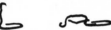

Start in the Padmasana posture and, with the help of the elbows, lower the trunk backward until, with the chest arching upwards, the top of the head is resting on the floor. Grasp the toes. Breathe lightly and avoid even the slightest tension.

Therapeutic effect: Overcomes any stiffness of the neck. The blood flowing out of the heart meets strong opposition, collects in the neck, and thoroughly cleanses the thyroid, the tonsils and the adenoids. Excellent for colds and purulent tonsils.

37. *Mayurasana**

Kneel on the floor, knees apart, palms down on the floor, fingers towards the feet, and squat on the heels. Bend forward and touch the floor with the forehead to obtain balance, and

155

then raise the feet and stretch the legs out behind. Raise the
head so that the body is supported only by the arms. A difficult
exercise which requires long practice.

Therapeutic effect: Excellent for equilibrium. Cleanses and
regenerates the digestive organs.

38. *Natapadasana*

After a certain age we neglect our posture and because we are
lazy and prefer the easy solution, we shall soon get used to
having a round back. Fatigue in the back and low backache is
caused by a hollow back. This exercise strengthens the spine
and relieves strain on the small of the back. Lie flat on the
back and raise the legs vertically, keeping the small of the back
on the ground. Inhaling, bring down the right leg to the right
side to touch the ground. Exhaling, raise again vertically.
Repeat with the left leg to the left.   3 ×

39. *Natarajasana*

An excellent exercise for balance and concentration.
Stand on the right leg, hold the left foot with the
left hand and lean slightly forward stretching the
right arm in front. Hold this position for a few
seconds with very relaxed breathing. Repeat with
the right leg.   3 ×

40. *Natashira-Vajrasana*

This exercise develops our resolution and sense of stability. Sit
on the heels with the hands on the knees. Breathing deeply,
raise the arms above the head, straighten up to stand on the

knees. While exhaling and kneeling, lean back as far as possible (do not bend but lean back). Inhaling, return to former kneeling position. Exhale and sit on the heels with hands on the knees.

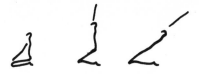

41. *Paschimotanasana**

Lie on the back and raise the arms while inhaling deeply until the arms are flat on the floor beside the body. Breathing calmly, sit up slowly, bending forward until the fingers touch the toes or until the ankles can be grasped. The knees must remain completely stiff. Bend the head forward until it touches the knees and rest the elbows on the floor. While breathing in deeply again, we sit up and lie back slowly on the floor, the arms at rest next to the body. Exhale and relax.

Therapeutic effect: Excellent for the abdominal organs. Reduces fat round the waist.

42. *Padahastasana**

The same as paschimotanasana but standing.

43. *Padangustasana*

To develop our power of concentration and introspection. Sitting on tiptoe with hands touching the ground on either side of the body, place the left foot on the right thigh while sitting on the right heel. With relaxed breathing raise the hands sideways to just below shoulder level. Repeat with the other leg.   3 ×

44. *Parshva-Bhunamanasana*

Sit with legs wide apart, hands clasped behind the back. Inhale deeply. While exhaling bend over the left leg to touch the knee with the forehead. Inhale deeply, sit upright, exhaling bend over the right leg. Inhale, sit upright and exhale, relax.   3 ×

Therapeutic effect: In addition to strengthening the spine, the proper functioning of the inner organs is stimulated.

45. *Parshva-Pada-calanasana*

Lying flat on the back raise the legs vertically with the arms stretched alongside the body. Inhale, while exhaling bring down both legs to the right side to touch the ground. Inhaling, raise the legs vertically, while exhaling bring legs down to left side.   3 ×

Therapeutic effect: Strengthens the legs and increases resolution.

46. *Parvatasana* (Mountain Pose)

Sit with legs crossed or on the heels. Inhale, place palms together directly above the head. Retaining the breath, stretch arms high above the head. Remain in this position for about 7 sec. Exhaling, place hands on the knees. Perform three times consecutively then rest.   3 ×

Therapeutic effect: Raises our will-power and power of resistance.

47. *Pavanamuktasana*

Lie on the back and hold the knees gently. Inhale deeply, when exhaling draw the knees tightly together with the hands. Inhale, relax the hold on the knees, when exhaling draw them tightly together. Do this about ten times consecutively. Stretch the legs and rest.   3 ×

Therapeutic effect: Because the blood is pressed out when the knees are drawn together, then allowed to gush in when inhaling with a relaxed hold on the knees, this unusually vigorous

158

massage regenerates all the inner organs. Constipation, a disorder which poisons and thus causes degeneration of the body,
is completely cured. Likewise diabetes and kidney troubles.

48. *Pavanamuktasana* (Sitting)

Sit on the ground and hold the knees gently. Inhale deeply and
relax the hold on the knees; exhaling, draw them tightly
together. Repeat seven to ten times consecutively. Rest with
hands and head on knees.

49. *Spine-strengthening exercises*

(*a*) Sit with the knees drawn up, the hands behind the back on
the ground. Now raise the hips as high as possible and slowly
walk ten steps forward on all fours (feet first) and ten steps back
again. After a short rest with deep breathing, repeat the
movement.

Therapeutic effect: 'The body is living when the tenant is alive.'
This movement on all fours brings the back and every single
muscle into motion. The result is that consciousness is led into
every part of the back, the arms, the legs and the chest. The
body becomes incredibly supple, conscious and is always
relaxed.

(*b*) A variation of this exercise is to lean forward and place the
palms on the ground, then to walk round the room on all fours,
if possible with stiff knees.

50. *Salabhasana**

Lie face down with the nose and forehead touching the floor

and place the fist on the floor beside the thighs. Make a full inhalation, retain the breath, and by pushing the fists against the floor, raise the outstretched legs as high as possible. After remaining like this a few moments, return to the original position and exhale.

Therapeutic effect: Excellent for preventing constipation, cleanses the kidneys and strengthens the spine.

51. *Sarpasana*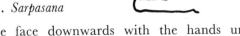

Lie face downwards with the hands under the forehead. During inhalation clasp the hands together behind the body with the arms extended and raise the head, chest and extended arms as high as possible.
Remain in this position for 3–5 sec and then return to the initial position, breathing out at the same time.

Therapeutic effect: Strengthens each vertebra, particularly the small of the back, the thorax and the upper back. Keeps the body elastic.

52. *Sarvangasana**

Lie on the back with the arms extended next to the body, palms on the floor. Slowly inhale and lift the extended legs without bending the knees until the legs are vertical above the body. As soon as this position is reached, raise the trunk so that the hips rest upon the hands. From here push the trunk upward until it and the legs are in a straight vertical line. The chin is pressed firmly against the chest. Breathe abdominally and remain in this posture as long as it is comfortable.

160

Therapeutic effect: Relaxes the heart, calms and strengthens the thyroid. Rejuvenates the entire system.

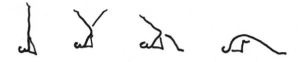

53. *Sarvangasana* (Variation)

Lying on the back and exhaling, raise legs and hips vertically, in candle posture, hold the hips with the hands. With relaxed breathing touch the ground with the right foot, the right knee well flexed. Repeat with the left leg. After two to three times come down and rest. 3 ×

When you have mastered this, try with all due caution when the right foot is on the ground to bring the left foot also to the ground. Hold the waist with the hands. After some seconds raise the right leg vertically again and then the left leg. Come down and rest.

Therapeutic effect: The heavy pressure on the kidney region thoroughly cleanses the kidneys of noxious waste matter.

54. *Savasana**

Lie on the back with both arms extended near the body. The feet are together and the legs stretched out to full length. Without exertion slow down the breathing as much as possible. Beginning with the feet relax all muscles. Withdraw consciousness to the heart. One minute of this active rest is equal to one hour of sleep.

Therapeutic effect: The nervous system gets complete rest. Best exercise for insomnia.

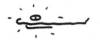

55. *Simhasana**

Sit with the legs crossed or on the heels, the hands resting on the knees. Exhaling, mouth open, stretch out the tongue as far as possible. When inhaling press the lower part of the tongue (tongue rolled) strongly up against the palate.　　　7–10 ×

Therapeutic effect: One of the most effective exercises to combat colds, throat troubles and tonsilitis as it causes vigorous blood circulation in the throat. Those who tax their throats such as teachers and singers will find this exercise extremely useful. The voice is crystal-clear.

56. *Sirshasana**

Kneel, interlacing the fingers, and placing the hands on the floor in front. Lean forward and place the head on the floor with the interlaced fingers supporting its back. With the help of the feet raise the hips up in the air. Then also lift the feet and bend the knees until equilibrium is obtained standing on the head. Slowly straighten the legs until the entire body is in a straight vertical line.

Therapeutic effect: Nourishes the brain and maintains mental health.

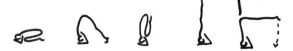

57. *Stambhasana*

Sit with the knees drawn up, hands behind the back on the ground. Raise the legs vertically and breathe slowly. After 20–30 sec rest with hands and forehead on the knees.　　　3 ×

Therapeutic effect: Enhances our will-power and powers of concentration and increases our resolution.

58. Supta-Vajrasana*

Kneel on the floor with the feet apart, lowering the body until a sitting posture between the heels is attained. With the aid of the arms and elbows, lower the trunk until the back of the head touches the floor. Place the hands behind the neck. Breathe without effort and direct the consciousness to the solar plexus and the heart.

Therapeutic effect: A highly stimulating exercise for a dull nervous system and underactive glandular functions.

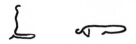

59. Tadaghi-Mudra

Lie flat on the back. Inhaling, raise the arms above the head, exhaling, sit up, bend forward and hold the ankles. Remaining without breath, draw the stomach in deeply. After 5–7 sec inhale deeply, lie flat on the back and rest.   3 ×

Therapeutic effect: Because the entire abdominal region is pressed together, the abdomen is directly massaged. It is also indirectly massaged when we draw it in deeply. This exercise helps to raise our inner power of resistance and the developed gastric fire clears a sluggish stomach, liver and particularly intestines. Highly effective against excess acid in the stomach, gall-stones and kidney-stones. Psychic effects are increased introspection and an exceptional power of concentration.

60. Trataka

Sit with crossed legs and fix your gaze on a small spot on the wall before you. Keeping the eyes wide open, with each breath lead, or rather, draw vital force directly into the eyes. Only when the eyes start burning close them for a moment and continue the exercise. Keep the eyes open for as long as possible without blinking. With a little practice you will be able to keep the eyes open for 5 min without blinking.

Therapeutic effect: Through regular, conscious breathing, prana (vital force) is directed into the eyes through the nerves which activate the eyes. Oxygen-saturated blood will circulate through the arteries from the centre to the periphery and remove toxins. This exercise is the quickest way to regenerate the eyes. That is why—in the experience of Yogis—it cures every kind of eye complaint. The exercise also increases introspection and gives us superiority and confidence.

61. *Trikonasana**

Standing with feet apart, raise the arms sideways, palms upwards, as far as shoulder height. Throughout the exercise hold the arms out in a straight line with the shoulders. While raising the arms, make a full Yoga inhalation. While exhaling, bend the trunk to the right and touch the right toes with the fingers of the right hand. Now stretch the arms vertically and turn the face upward. On straightening up, inhale and then, with only a moment's pause, slowly bend to the left and exhale. After a short pause, straighten up again while inhaling, then slowly lower the arms sidewards while breathing out. Consciousness is held in the spine.

Therapeutic effect: Affords lateral exercise for the backbone.

62. *Trikonasana* (Variation)

(*a*) Stand upright with feet together. Inhale deeply. When exhaling, bend forward with the head held high up, and with the fingertips, touch the toes. Remain in this position for some seconds without drawing a breath. Inhaling deeply, return to the upright position and exhale. Remain standing and rest.   3 ×

Therapeutic effect: Vigorous blood circulation in the hips and back removes any fatty deposits. The psychic effect is an upright state of mind and self-reliance.

(*b*) Stand upright with legs apart. Inhaling deeply, raise arms to shoulder level, the palms facing upward. While exhaling touch the left foot with the right hand, simultaneously turning the upper body far over to the left. Inhale standing upright with arms stretched to the sides. Exhale touching the right foot with the left hand turning the upper body to the right. Inhale standing upright, exhale and lower arms, palms facing downward.   3 ×

(*c*) Stand upright with legs apart. Exhaling, touch the left foot with the right hand, simultaneously strongly flexing the left knee. The left arm is stretched above the head and held parallel to the ground. After 5 sec inhale, returning to the upright position with stretched, raised arms. Exhaling, touch the right foot with the left hand, at the same time strongly flexing the right knee. The right arm is stretched above the head and held parallel to the ground. After 5 sec inhale deeply returning to the upright position with stretched, raised arms, exhaling, lower the arms and rest.   3 ×

Therapeutic effect: Exercises the spine laterally. The side muscles of the trunk are alternately tautened and relaxed. The trunk stretches to the right and to the left thereby bringing into play the entire set of back muscles supporting the vertebrae. The side muscles and the spine are vitalised. The vertebrae are subjected to lateral pressure and tension. Through this the spine receives the necessary elasticity and is brought into the right relation with the hip bones and muscular system. Complete recovery is accelerated after infectious illnesses as toxins lingering in the organism are made to dissolve. Numerous latent infections are removed from the body.

63. *Uddiyana-Bandha**

Stand with feet apart and trunk bent slightly forward, holding the arms straight and placing the hands upon the slightly bent knees. After a full Yoga inhalation, slowly exhale and draw the abdominal wall in tight by raising the diaphragm as high as possible.

Therapeutic effect: Stimulates the intestines.

64. *Uddiyana-Bandha* (Squatting)

Inhale deeply in squatting position. After exhaling forcefully draw in the abdomen deeply. Remain without breath for 7–10 sec. Inhale deeply and rest.   3 ×

65. *Uddiyana-Bandha* (Variation)

Stand upright with legs apart. Inhale deeply. After exhaling forcefully draw in the abdomen deeply, stretch the arms at a slant above the head so that the arms and legs form an X. Inhale deeply, exhale and lower arms from the front, rest.   3 ×

Therapeutic effect: Through the strong contraction of the diaphragm, the organs of the abdominal cavity are given an exceptional indirect massage. Extremely effective against collapse of the stomach, kidneys, and, in the case of women, the womb. Furthers the transformation or sublimation of sexual energies. Recommended for adolescents and young men with frequent ejaculations. Excellent for fatty deposits on abdomen and hips. Improves the digestion.

66. *Urdva-Paschimotanasana*

Sit with the knees tucked in. Hold the ankles with the hands and stretch the legs up vertically. Breathing out and keeping the legs vertical, touch the knees with the forehead. After 5 sec rest with the knees tucked in.   3 ×

Therapeutic effect: The tremendous pressure exerted on the abdominal region presses out a large quantity of blood from the internal organs. When the body returns to the position of rest, oxygen-saturated blood suddenly gushes into the great blood vessels called arcus aortae and aorta abdominalis. The stomach, the liver, the spleen, the kidneys and the intestines are strengthened and regenerated. Every disorder, ailment and disease of these organs is cured. This exercise is highly recommended for diabetics. The pancreas gland is brought under control.

67. *Ustrasana* (Camel Posture)

Sit on the heels, feet together. Holding the ankles with both hands, raise the small of the back and pelvis as high as possible. Breathing deeply, remain in this position for 5–10 sec. Sitting on the heels lean forward, place the head on the fists and rest.   3 ×

68. *Uttha-Janusirasana*

Stand upright with feet together. Inhale deeply. While exhaling, raise outstretched right leg, simultaneously exhaling and bending forward to hold the ankle. Try to touch the right knee with the forehead. Then inhale while lowering the leg and straighten up. Exhale repeating the process with the left leg. Rest awhile, breathing slowly and deeply.   3 ×

Therapeutic effect: Strengthens all the muscles of the back and legs. Gives self-confidence and self-reliance.

69. *Vajrasana* (Diamond posture)

Sit on the heels. Lean back and place the elbows on the ground behind the body. Hold the hips with the hands and raise them as high as possible. At the same time drop the head backward to touch the ground. Breathe regularly. After a time bend

forward and rest, the head supported by the fists. After some
practice the abdomen and hips remain raised to form a bridge.
When you can do this, try to place the hands on the thighs. 3 ×

Therapeutic effect: As the name implies, this exercise gives the
body the resilient toughness of a diamond. The circulation is
restricted in the lower part of the body, but is all the more
vigorous in the organs of the abdominal cavity, in the chest,
the thyroid gland, the face and the brain. Excellent for breathing difficulties and heart troubles. Fatigue of eyes and brain
quickly disappears. Improves the eyesight.

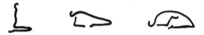

70. *Vajroli-Mudra*

Sit with the knees tucked in, palms before you on the
ground. Raise the legs up, breathing regularly. After
about 20 sec tuck in the knees and rest with hands and
forehead on the knees.   3 ×

Therapeutic effect: This exercise raises our will-power
and power of resistance and at the same time increases
perseverance and resolution.

71. *Vakrasana**

Sit on the floor with the legs stretched out in front. Draw up
the right leg so that the thigh and the knee are pressed hard
against the abdomen and chest. Lift the right foot over the left
and place the sole of the right foot next to the left thigh on the
floor. The palms of both hands are placed flat on the floor,
fingers outward. After three full Yoga breathings, change feet
and repeat.

168

Therapeutic effect: The positive and negative currents are brought into equilibrium.

72. *Vakrasana* (Variation)

Sit with the legs wide apart. Inhale deeply, stretching the arms above the head, keeping the palms together. Exhale turning the upper body slowly to the right. Inhale turning the body to the front, exhale slowly turning to the left, inhaling, turn to the front again, exhale and rest with the hands on the knees.   3 ×

Therapeutic effect: The important nerve centres in the spine are charged with vital force, whereby fatigue and nervousness are eliminated.

73. *Vibhakta-Janusirasana*
See No. 27: Hastapadasana

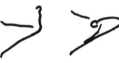

74. *Viparita-Karani**

Lie on the back and slowly inhale. Raise the legs upward and, supporting the hips with the hands, gradually raise the trunk until it is resting on the shoulder-blades. The legs and feet are inclined slightly beyond the head. Remain in this posture as long as it is comfortable and maintained without undue exertion.

Therapeutic effect: Very similar to Sarvangasana.

75. *Viparita-Karani* (Variation)

Lying on the back, raise up the legs and hold the hips
with the hands. Breathe regularly. Gradually stretch the
body until you are standing on the shoulders and hold
the knees with the hands. Hold this position for up to
1 min, then rest lying on the back with relaxed breathing.   3 ×

Therapeutic effect: The thyroid glands are calmed and
strengthened. The nerve cells in the brain are quickly
charged. Excellent for varicose veins.

76. *Vrksasana*

Stand upright. Place the left foot on the right thigh or
on the right knee. Stretch the arms above the head
with the palms together. Breathe regularly. After 30 sec
change over, that is to say, place the right foot on the
left thigh.   3 ×

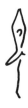

Therapeutic effect: An excellent exercise for physical and mental
balance which develops one's power of concentration.

77. *Vrksasana* (Tree posture) Variation

Sit on the heels with the palms on the ground beside the knees.
Place the head on a soft cushion before you and stretch the
knees. Raise the legs one after the other from the ground until
you are standing on the head. Breathe regularly. After about
30 sec sit on the heels again. Bend forward and rest with the
forehead on the fists.   3 ×

Those with any kind of spinal infirmity must not perform this
exercise.

Therapeutic effect: Strengthens the vertebral column. Offers relief for the brain. Increases the sense of equilibrium, both physically and mentally.

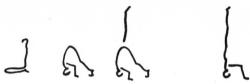

78. *Yastikasana* (Stick posture)

Lie flat on the back. Inhaling deeply, stretch the arms above the head on the ground. Retaining the breath, stretch the body from fingertips to toes, as hard as possible. After 10–20 sec, exhale lowering the arms down to the sides. Rest. 3 ×

Therapeutic effect: Excellent for those with back trouble as each vertebra is stretched and relaxed. Those with sedentary occupations should perform this exercise daily.

79. *Yoga-Mudra* (With fists on the abdomen)

Sitting on the heels, inhale deeply. While exhaling, press the abdomen with the fists and bend forward to the ground. Remain without taking a breath for about 10 sec. Sitting up, inhale deeply. Exhale and place the hands on the knees. 3 ×

Therapeutic effect: Intense pressure on the abdomen removes the blood from this region. When returning to the upright position the vigorous circulation regenerates all the organs of the abdominal cavity.

80. *Yoga-Mudra* (Variation)

Performed exactly as the previous exercise, with the one difference that the arms are raised vertically behind the body, the hands clasped. 3 ×

81. *Yoga-Mudra* (Variation)

Sitting on the heels, inhale, but only half fill the lungs. Retaining the breath bend forward to the ground. Keep the hands together behind the body. After 10 sec sit up and only then exhale.   3 ×

*Exercises marked with an asterisk are discussed at greater length and in many cases illustrated in *Yoga and Health* (S. Yesudian and E. Haich, Unwin Books).

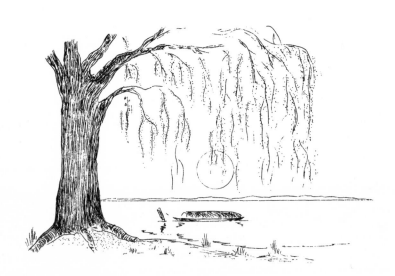

5 Meditation

Maintain a state of tranquillity in all your actions: a calm man can achieve anything. Life can be enjoyed better when we are the masters of our warring senses, not their slaves. Only when the outgoing forces are brought under control do we become aware of the creative forces at our disposal and the potential strength we possess. The man who is strong is fearless. Enjoying the attributes of strength and fearlessness he is free to act and live in the world as he likes.

This state is easily attained through the practice of meditation. Start and close the day with meditation, devoting about 10–15 min daily to this habit of turning the mind within, and later it will continue all day, helping you to discriminate in all matters.

Just as food is given to the body, so good impressions should be put into the subconscious mind. Read the teachings of Buddha, Jesus, Ramakrishna, Vivekananda, Ramana Maharshi, etc. In time this habit will create an atmosphere of peace and purity around you wherever you go.

HOW TO MEDITATE

Sit on the ground on a cushion with legs crossed; or on your heels on a rug; or, should this be uncomfortable, on a chair. Drop the shoulders but keep the back upright. Place palms on the knees. Maintain a normal rhythm of breathing. BE THE STATE OF PERFECT PEACE. Turn the mind within and be identified with your SELF. Repeat mentally: 'I am not the body nor the mind nor the feelings. I am neither sight nor speech nor hearing nor taste. I am not the five senses. The body is the outer covering of the SELF which is pure and perfect. I am the boundless, the limitless, the deathless spirit. I am the ever-free. I am the eternal present. I AM WHO I AM.'

The repetition of these thoughts will enable you to train your mind to obey you. Unless you check the mind, the senses will drag you down. These thoughts are only essential at the beginning, for later the trained mind will follow the right direction. With introspection the mind becomes steady. Discrimination begins when you are able to clearly see the difference between the essential and the non-essential, truth and untruth, virtue and vice, etc. 'In a conflict between the head and the heart, choose the heart,' said Vivekananda. Meditation is the only means of learning to discriminate. This daily habit will help you to choose the essential. He who is in possession of truth has found peace and happiness.

Meditation will in time be a normal state even during work. Though we live in this world and perform our duties, our heart will always be at peace. Thus work and wisdom will be the same.

6 More Guiding Thoughts of the Great Masters and Thoughts and Poems by the Author

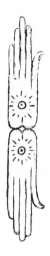

Sanctified was the day of my birth, and
Sanctified my stay on earth shall be.

S.Y.

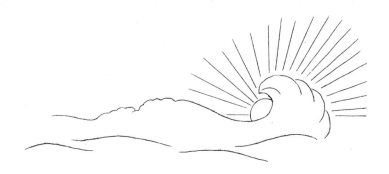

To succeed, you must have tremendous perseverance,
tremendous will. 'I will drink the ocean,' says the per-
severing soul. 'At my will mountains will crumble.' Have
that sort of energy, that sort of will, work hard, and you
will reach the goal.

Vivekananda

Disciple: I value my individuality however unimportant it may be. I do not wish to be absorbed into this eternal unity. The mere thought fills me with horror.

Vivekananda answered: One day a drop of water fell into the ocean. When it realised what had happened it began to weep and complain as you are doing now. The giant ocean laughed at the tiny drop of water. 'Why are you crying?' it asked. 'I cannot understand. Just as you have become one with me, so you have become one with your brothers and sisters, the other drops of water of which I consist. You too will be the ocean itself. If you want to leave me, ascend into the clouds on a sunbeam. From there, tiny drop of water, you can descend again to bless the thirsting earth.'

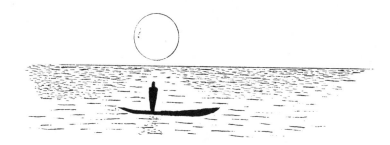

Regard your mother as God. Regard your father as God.
Regard your teacher as God.

Kathopanishad

We should be Christians as regards mercy, Mohammedans
as regards strict observance of external rules and Hindus
as regards love of all living creatures.

Ramakrishna

You must be dead, as it were, to all arrogance, illusions
of grandeur and vanity.

Swami Sabhapatti

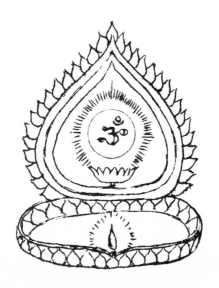

The healthy individual raises the value of the whole nation, for as a part of the whole he forms the whole. We need calm, peaceable, healthy and strong men. They alone can do good deeds and achieve a lasting, beneficial effect. We need men whose energies have not been squandered but stored up and held in check.

S.Y.

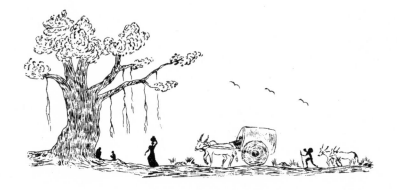

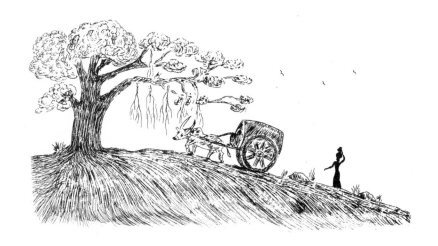

He indeed is blessed in whom all the qualities of head and heart are fully developed and evenly balanced. He bears himself well in whatever position he may be placed. He is full of guileless faith and love for God, and yet his dealings with others leave nothing to be desired. When he engages in worldly affairs he is a thorough man of business; in the assembly of the learned, he establishes his claims as a man of learning, and in debates, he shows great powers of reasoning. To his parents he is obedient and affectionate; to his brethren and friends he is loving and sweet; to his neighbours he is kind and sympathetic, always ready to do good; and to his wife he is the lord of love. Such a man is indeed perfect.

Sri Ramakrishna

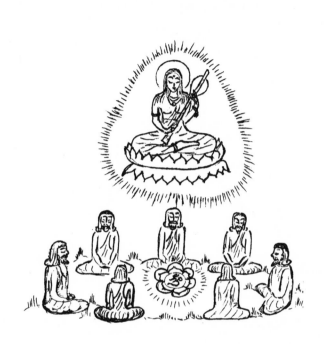

The Revelation of the Vedas

Lakshmana once said to his Divine brother, 'Is it not strange, O Rama, that a Jnani (an initiate) like Vasishtha Deva should have wept for the loss of his sons, and would not be comforted?'

Rama replied, 'True, my brother, but bear in mind that whoever possesses Jnana (wisdom) must at the same time have Ajnana (ignorance) also; whoever has the knowledge of unity must also have the knowledge of diversity; whoever has the consciousness of light must have the consciousness of darkness also; because all these, being correlatives, belong to the domain of nescience. Unless one goes beyond both of them, one cannot be free from sorrow and ignorance.'

Sri Ramakrishna

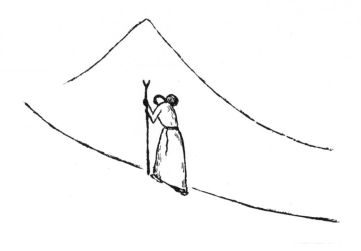

Alone I wander, with no home
to claim me as her own.
Alone I wander, with naught
to claim as my own.
On the endless shores of creation I stand
to claim all as my own.

S.Y.

The Village Where I was Born

Something calls in the depths of my heart,
    What could it be, I wonder?
A voice which calls both night and day,
    It speaks of my birthplace yonder.
It lies beyond the seven seas,
    Beyond the great blue mountains,
A little house of mud and stone
    Beside two little fountains.

It tells me of my childhood days,
    Of my dreams, my joys and fun,
How I wandered alone from dawn to dusk,
    Not a soul did I meet, not one.
The paddy fields were rich and green
    By the black granite hill,
And from the hill-top I did scan
    The village beneath so still.

Often I heard the temple bells
    Calling to even-song
The humble peasants in the field
    Who work the whole day long.
Again I hear her chiming voice
    Calling her far-off son,
As she did when I sat on a mountain-top:
    'Come home, my little one.'

                                    S.Y.

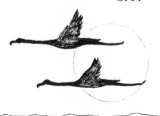

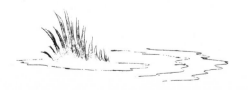

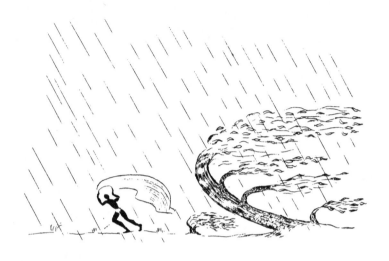

That which has form and attributes is also without form
and attributes. God (Brahma) and his power (Shakti) are
not separate entities, but rather, the one divine principle
under the two aspects of the masculine and the feminine.

Ramakrishna

The man whose energies are dissipated lacks peace. The
man who concentrates is calm and superior, for his
energies are gathered together. Practise meditation daily.
It will rouse your dormant abilities. If the energies are
concentrated, any task can be accomplished.

S.Y.

Freedom means: to be free of all illusions.

Vivekananda

D.: What is the best time of day for meditation?
M.: What is time?

Ramana Maharshi

He who perceives the goal cannot lose the way.

S.Y.

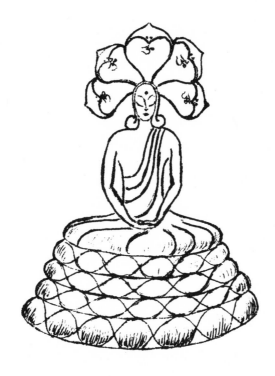

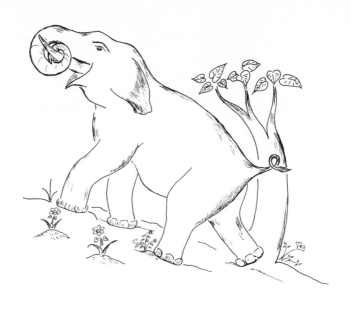

Go forward without a path!
Fearing nothing, caring for nothing!
Wander alone, like a rhinoceros!
Even as the lion not trembling at noises,
Even as the wind not caught in the net,
Even as the lotus leaf, unstained by the water,
Do thou wander alone like the rhinoceros!

Dhammapada

Leave this chanting and singing and telling of beads!
Whom dost thou worship in this lonely dark corner of a
    temple with doors all shut?
Open thine eyes and see thy God is not before thee!

He is there where the tiller is tilling the hard ground
and where the pathmaker is breaking stones.
He is with them in sun and in shower,
and his garment is covered with dust.
Put off thy holy mantle and even like him
come down on the dusty soil!

Deliverance? Where is this deliverance to be found?
Our master himself has joyfully
taken upon him the bonds of creation;
he is bound with us all for ever.

Come out of thy meditations
and leave aside thy flowers and incense!
What harm is there if thy clothes
become tattered and stained?
Meet him and stand by him
in toil and in the sweat of thy brow.

Rabindranath Tagore

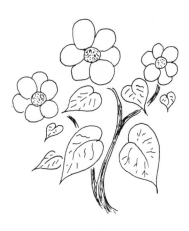

People talk of enjoying this world, but do they know how? First become a God and then enjoy. Before that, all your enjoyments are the enjoyments of a brute.

Brahmananda.

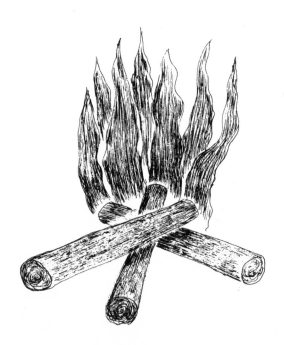

When blinding passions rage within my being,
Let me but raise the sails
To catch their carrying winds.
And on their waters deep with mountain waves,
May I speed straight without a stop
To the horizon of my dream,
Past passion's night,
From darkness into light.
From blackness of night,
Into dawn's glory of light.

S.Y.

The babbling brooks and singing streams
race down into the river, only to end in their
endless ocean home. So I race on to Thee,
through the hill and dale of thy creation,
until breaking through all barriers,
  I join Thee, the endless.
  I join Thee, the eternal.
  I join Thee, the everlasting.

S.Y.

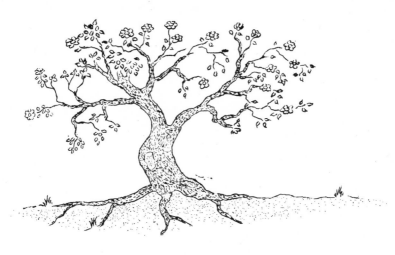

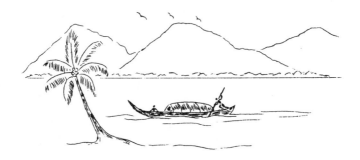

It is impossible to see God, the begetter of the universe, with our mortal eyes. God is spirit and we can only be spirit. Religion shows us the way to this. True religion is therefore the realisation of the spirit.

S.Y.

It is the aim of the Yogi to perfect himself, and in so doing he attains spiritual bliss.

S.Y.

If your freedom hurts others, you are not free. You must not hurt others.

Vivekananda

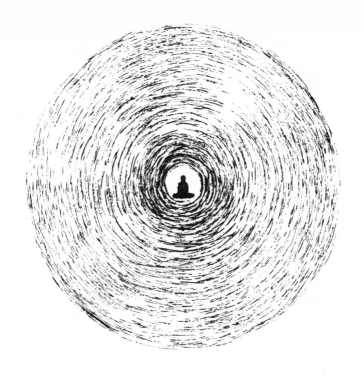

S: I cannot control my mind.
R: Why not? There is something called Abhyasoyoga,
which means Yoga through practice. Practise regularly
and you will see that your mind follows wherever you
may guide it. The mind is like white cloth that comes
from the cleaner's. It turns red if you dye it in red, and
blue if you dye it in blue. It will assume whatever colour
you choose.

Ramakrishna

Just as the path of the eagle in the air and the path of the snake are invisible, so also is the path of the sage.

Buddha

'Oh Arjuna! I have no duty in the whole wide world,' says Krishna. Be perfectly resigned, perfectly unconcerned, only then can you do any true work.

Vivekananda

There are two things which always remain the same: good deeds bring inner peace and happiness, bad ones bring spiritual chaos and despair.

Buddha

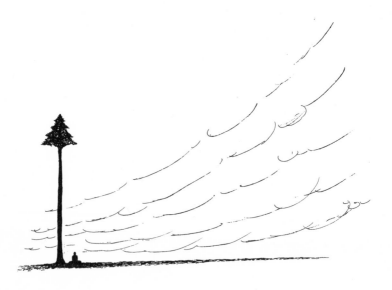

Long is the night to him who is awake; long is a mile to him who is tired; long is life to the foolish who do not know the true law.

If a traveller does not meet with one who is his better, or his equal, let him firmly keep to his solitary journey; there is no companionship with a fool.

The fool who knows his foolishness, is wise at least so far. But a fool who thinks himself wise, he is called a fool indeed.

Fools of poor understanding have themselves for their greatest enemies, for they do evil deeds which bear bitter fruits.

That deed is not well done of which a man must repent, and the reward of which he receives crying and with a tearful face. No, that deed is well done of which a man does not repent, and the reward of which he receives gladly and cheerfully.

Buddha

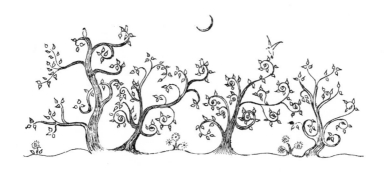

Tear down the veil that blinds thy sight,
That dims thy mind, holding thy tongue a captive.
Speak out thy freedom
With a fearless breath
And break the bonds of time.
Eternity thy goal!
No prisoner more
To crawl below the senses' heavy lash.
Burst asunder thy chains of love or hate,
For both do bind.
And raise thy lion head
To look around the wide expanse
Of eternal freedom ever thine.

S.Y.

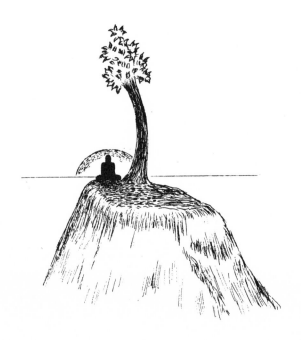

The Beggar's Rags

I have run miles and passed by many milestones all this way, and I have hurried to be in time for the feast of which Thou hast summoned me to partake, O my Master.

As a beggar I waited with empty hands. Now, with speechless lips, I stand amazed and bewildered at the wealth that lies before my feet.

Thou dost give, but my pockets are tattered and torn, and I know not where to put this gold. Now, with a touch of Thy tender love my poverty doth cease, and instead of rags my garments are of gold.

I would play on my wooden flute, but joy doth flood this heart of mine.
So now in silence let me wander this garden and end my days in peaceful prayer.

S.Y.

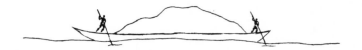

Religion is to go beyond everything that is human in us and to touch the divine. Where else is this attainable if not within?

S.Y.

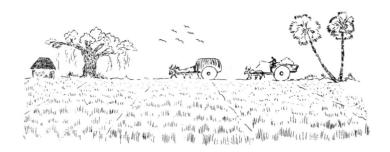

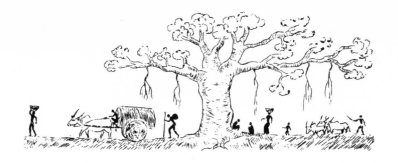

With increasing resilience, suffering and disease disappear.
With the perception of the positive energies accumulated
in such a short time our outlook will become serene. A
calm frame of mind will greatly enable us to perform our
duties, because all our energies are gathered together.

S.Y.

I must manifest the highest. I cannot be satisfied with
anything less than the highest.

S.Y.

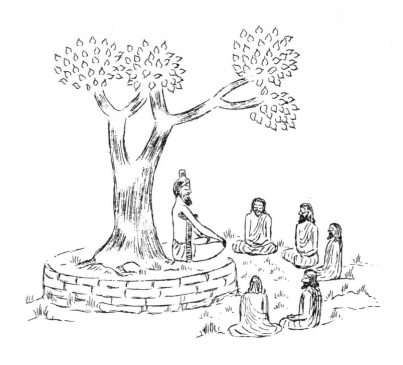

The test of the steadiness of mind is the steadiness of look. As soon as the mind becomes steady, the look also becomes steady. No more is there any restlessness in one's looks and movements.

Turiyananda

198

If a man has experienced suffering and knows the nature of suffering, how can he thoughtlessly inflict it on another?

The suffering which one man inflicts on another comes back to him that very afternoon.

The best punishment for those who treat us badly is to make them ashamed by rewarding bad with good.

Has humanity a greater enemy than anger which kills laughter and joy? (Which are truly the greatest blessings of this world.)

If people would see their own faults as they see those of others, then evil would soon be erased from this world.

If you are faithful in word and thought you are superior to him who does penance and offers sacrifices.

There is no greater wealth than an ungrudging nature.

Tiruvalluvar

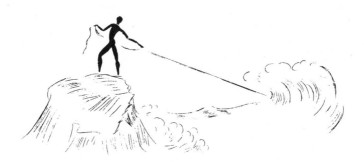

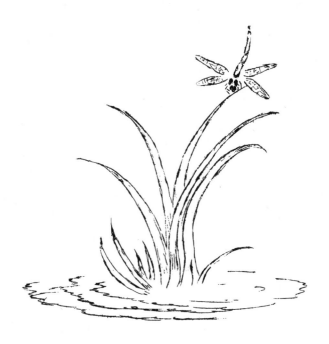

Learn to feel yourself in other bodies, to know that we are all one. Throw all other nonsense to the winds. Spit out your actions, good or bad, and never think of them again. What is done is done. Throw off superstition. Have no weakness even in the face of death. Do not repent, do not brood over past deeds, and do not remember your good deeds. Be free. The weak, the fearful, the ignorant will never reach the Self.

Vivekananda

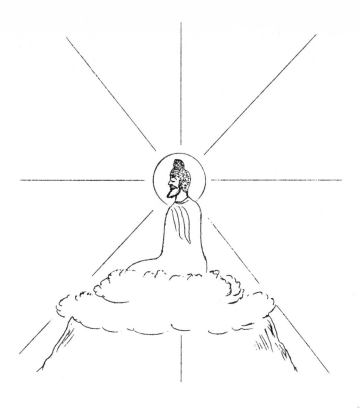

Arise! Awake! What are you doing? If the body is to go, let it go working. Rousing the divinity in yourself and in others—that is the ideal.

Vivekananda

By rousing himself, by earnestness, by restraint and control, the wise man can make for himself an island which no flood can sweep away.

Buddha

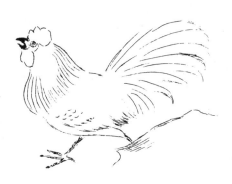

Friendship is not for pleasant laughter, but for harsh advice promptly to be given when one swerves from the right path.

Tiruvalluvar

It is true, Simba, that I denounce action, but only such action as leads to evil in thought, speech and deed. It is true, Simba, that I preach annihilation, but only the annihilation of pride, passion, evil thoughts and ignorance, never that of forgiveness, love, mercy, and truth.

Buddha

Enjoy the pleasure that is your lot and bear the sorrow that is your lot; await serenely that which time will bring, as the farmer awaits his crops.

Mahabharatam

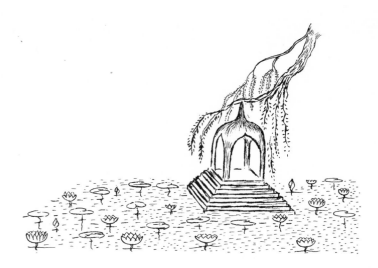

The man who gives way to anger, or hatred, or any other passion, cannot work, he only breaks himself to pieces, and does nothing practical. It is the calm, forgiving, equable, well-balanced mind that does the greatest amount of work.

Vivekananda

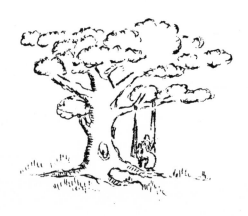

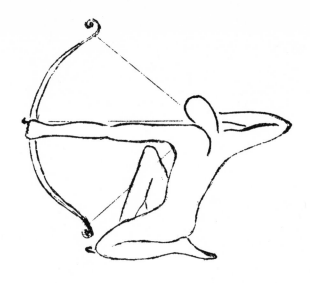

To survive is the law of nature. But cowards perish. They are mercilessly swept away by the current of circumstances. It is the hero who lives and enjoys the earth.

S.Y.

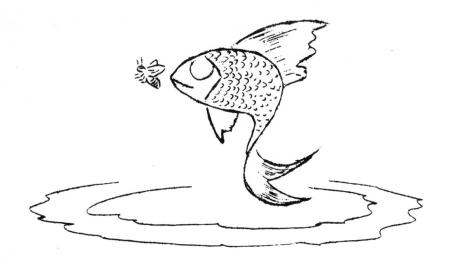

If atavism gains, you go down; if evolution gains, you
go on.

Vivekananda

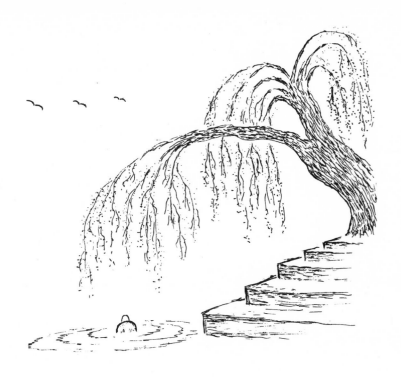

The means of destruction of ignorance is the unbroken practice of discrimination.

Patanjali

Familiarise yourself with the thought that you are spirit, conscious, free, fearless and strong. Know that the manifestation of this spirit depends on you.

S.Y.

Knowing that you are the Infinite, fear must die. Say ever, 'I and my Father are one.'

Vivekananda

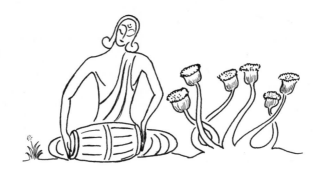

If Heaven created man, he must serve some purpose.

The infinite future is before you, and you must always remember that each word, thought and deed lays up store for you and that as the bad thoughts and bad works are ready to spring upon you like tigers, so also there is the inspiring hope that the good thoughts, and good deeds are ready with the power of a hundred thousand angels to defend you always and forever.

Vivekananda

Man is an all-powerful being. His experiences will one day awake the sleeping giant within him, at which he may rise up and testify to his own greatness and strength. Are not man's achievements evidence of his greatness and his boundless nature? Will he not always reach new heights? Has he already covered all the pages of the book of life with writing? Just as the heavens are immeasurable, so also are the potentialities of man.

S.Y.

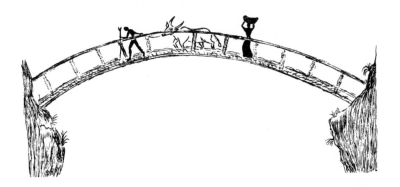

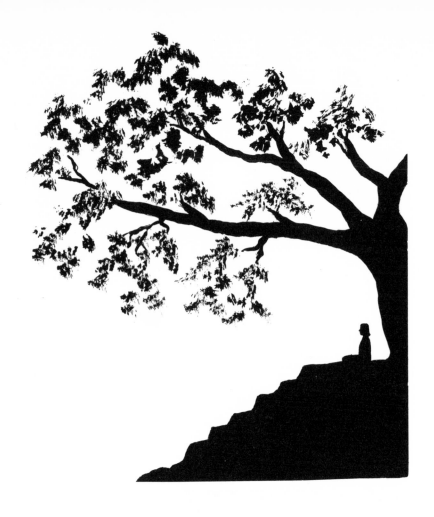

Buddha did not believe in power or anything of the kind. He spoke only of the annihilation of desires. He sat to meditate beneath a tree and said: 'Let this body dry away here', i.e. let me die on the spot if I cannot reach Nirvana. 'This body is a great rogue. Nothing can be achieved without controlling it.'

Vivekananda

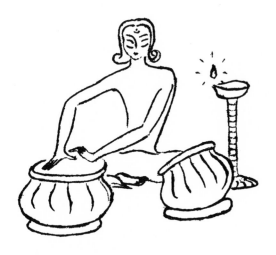

Learn the truth of the Divine Self only from those who themselves have realised it. From the others it would merely be idle prattle. Realisation is above virtue and vice, above future and past, above all alternatives. The pure and spotless man sees the SELF in everything and eternal peace reigns in his soul. Neither talk, discussion, reading of the Scriptures, highest flight of the intellect, nor even the Vedas are able to yield any knowledge of the Self.

Vivekananda

To my Muse

I have caught thine echo resounding in silent whispers from the depths of my fathomless soul.

I have seen thee play on the strings of my heart, the sad music of my soul caught in the meshes of this world.

And I have seen thee snap its strings and burst into a melody which only my freed soul could sing.

S.Y.

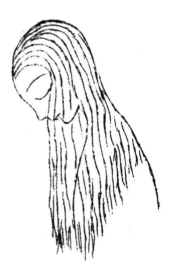

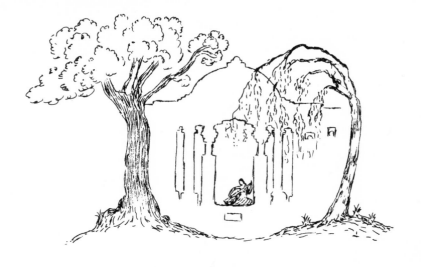

This is the only way to reach the goal, to tell ourselves,
and to tell everybody else, that we are divine. And as we
go on repeating this, strength comes. He who falters at
first will get stronger and stronger, and the voice will
increase in volume until the truth takes possession of our
hearts, and courses through our veins, and permeates our
bodies. Delusion will vanish as the light becomes more
and more effulgent, load after load of ignorance will
vanish, and then will come a time when all else has
disappeared and the sun alone shines.

Vivekananda

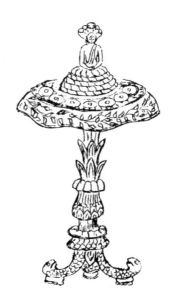

The more we conceal our religious practices from others, the better it is for ourselves.

Turn your thoughts to God in a quiet corner, in the forests or within yourself.

Fans are superfluous when the wind blows. We may cease prayers and penitential exercises when the grace of God descends.

He who has faith has everything, and he who lacks it lacks everything.

Sri Ramakrishna

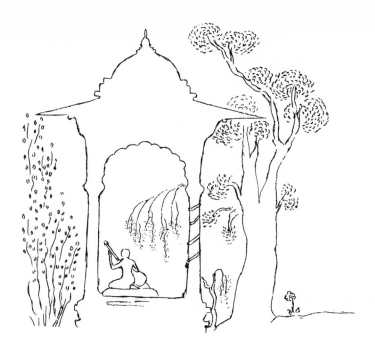

Concentration will bring perfect repose to mind and body
every time it is practised.

Vivekananda

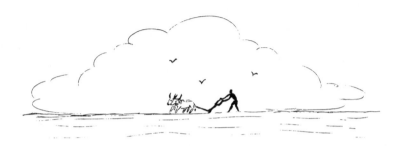

Q.: How should we live in this world?
A.: Perform all your duties, but dwell in God. Live with everyone—children, father and mother. Treat them as your intimate friends, but know that they do not belong to you.

Ramakrishna

'These sons belong to me, and this wealth belongs to me': with such thoughts a fool is tormented. He himself does not belong to himself; how much less sons and wealth?

Buddha

The body is my chariot, the five senses are my steeds, the intellect is my rein, but I AM THE CHARIOTEER.

Bhagavad Gita

He who has shaken off the fetters of time will do the best
work.

S.Y.

It is impossible to make progress as long as we still have
reason to feel shame, hatred and fear.

Ramakrishna

Only a cultured humanity can redeem the world.

Pestalozzi

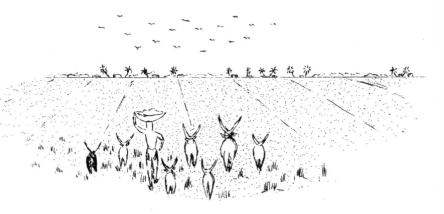

The Self is without parts and without a second; but the body is composed of many parts. And yet they court the two. Can any ignorance be worse than this?

The Self is the ruler and subjective; the body is the ruled and objective. And yet they court the two. Can any ignorance be worse than this?

The Self is of the nature of knowledge and is pure; the body consists of flesh and is impure. And yet they court the two. Can any ignorance be worse than this?

Sankaracharya

'All created things perish': he who knows and sees this becomes passive in pain; this is the way to purity.
'All created things are grief and pain': he who knows and sees this becomes passive in pain; this is the way to purity.

Buddha

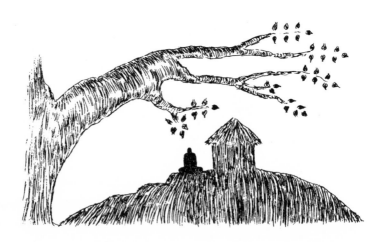

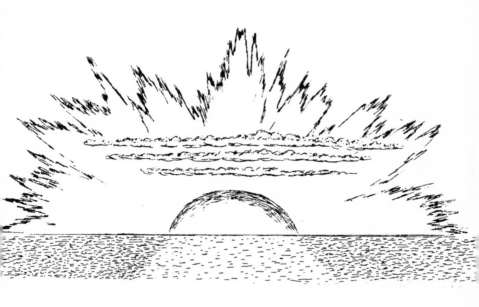

In Thine endless play of creation, Thou hast created me to play the game which knows no end. Such is Thy pleasure.

S.Y.

I slept and dreamt: life was joy.
I awoke and saw: life was duty.
I acted and saw: duty was joy.

Tagore

The journey before me is long. I have covered countless tracks and have wandered many a world. Drunk with the beauty of Thy creation I have slept on many a star.

S.Y.

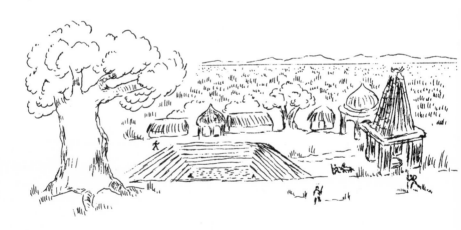

There are hundreds of thousands of teachers, but it is hard to find one disciple.

Indian wisdom

He alone is free who controls his urges and is not the slave of his passions, lusts and desires.

E. Haich

If aught there be that's mightier than Fate
'Tis courage that bears its blows uncowed.

Shakespeare

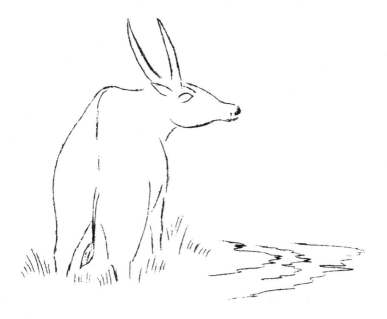

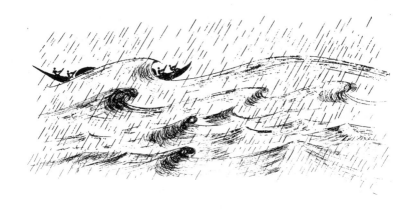

Look upon good and evil with an impartial eye. Then they cannot affect you. He who is not affected by good cannot be affected by evil.

S.Y.

In God's creation there can be nothing wrong. Learn to look upon suffering as part of God's plan. The ultimate outcome of suffering is always good.

S.Y.

As Arjuna raises his bow and aims, Drona asks: 'What do you see, Arjuna? Do you see the tree?'—'No, lord.'—'Do you see the branches?'—'No, lord.'—'Do you see the bird?'—'No, lord.' 'What do you see then, Arjuna?'— 'Oh noble lord, I see only the eye of the bird.' And who does not feel that he who worships similarly cannot see anything except God? And who is not absolutely certain that with such singleness of devotion the target 'God' must be reached?

S.Y.

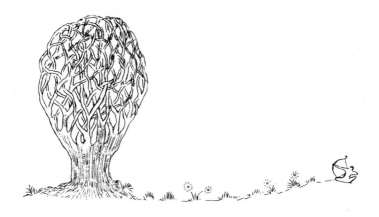

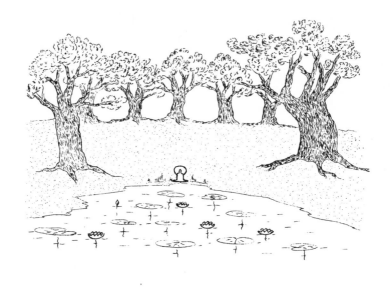

Q.: Is solitude necessary for a Jnani? (for one on the path of knowledge).

M.: Solitude is in the mind. One might be in the thick of the world and maintain serenity of mind; such a person is in solitude. Another may stay in a forest, but still be unable to control his mind. He cannot be said to be in solitude. Solitude is a function of the mind. A man attached to desire cannot find solitude wherever he may be; a detached man is always in solitude.

Sri Ramana Maharshi

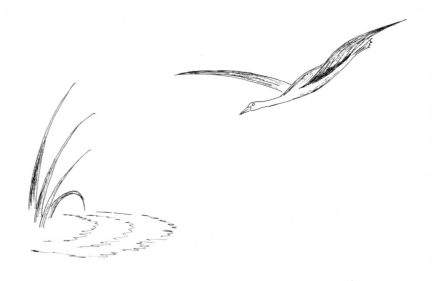

In one salutation to thee, my God, let all my senses spread out and touch this world at thy feet.

Like a rain-cloud of July hung low with its burden of unshed showers let all my mind bend down at thy door in one salutation to thee. Let all my songs gather together their diverse strains into a single current and flow to a sea of silence in one salutation to thee. Like a flock of home-sick cranes flying night and day back to their mountain nests, let all my life take its voyage to its eternal home in one salutation to thee.

Rabindranath Tagore

Life is merely a bridge. Do not build a house upon it.

Chinese wisdom

Revenge brings pleasure only for a day, patience brings
glory for all time.

Tiruvalluvar

Raise your heads, for each of you bears God within you.
Be worthy and proud of this.

Vedanta

Just as we cast off an old garment and put on a new one,
so the spirit clothed in the body will one day cast off its
old body and clothe itself in a new one.

Bhagavad Gita

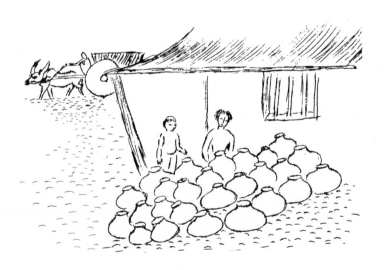

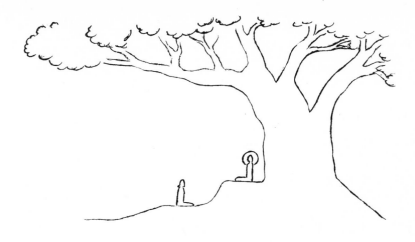

I saw the teacher sitting under a tree. He was a young
man of sixteen and the disciple was an old man of eighty.
The preaching of the teacher was silence, and the doubts
of the doubter departed.

He who thinks 'I am the body' remains, alas in ignorance, as also he who thinks 'this body is mine', as if he were always looking at an earthen vessel belonging to him.

'I am indeed Brahman (Spirit), without difference, without change, and of the nature of reality, knowledge and bliss. I am not, therefore, the body which is unreal.' This is what the wise call knowledge.

'I am without change, without form, without blemish and without decay. I am not, therefore, the body which is unreal.' This is what the wise call knowledge.

'I am without disease, without appearances, without alternatives, and all-pervading. I am not, therefore, the body which is unreal.' This is what the wise call knowledge.

'I am without attribute, without action, eternal, eternally free, and imperishable. I am not, therefore, the body which is unreal.' This is what the wise call knowledge.

'I am stainless, without motion, without end, pure, and devoid of old age and death. I am not, therefore, the body which is unreal.' This is what the wise call knowledge.

Sankaracharya

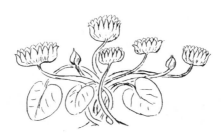

Prayer is not a passive approach asking God to fulfil our desires, but a time of deep introspection, discrimination, decision and intense action.

S.Y.

The SELF is not to be gained by the weak. If there is no strength in body and mind, the Self cannot be realised. First you have to build the body by good nutritious food— then only will the mind be strong. The mind is but the subtle part of the body. You must retain great strength in your mind and words.

Vivekananda

Materialism says the voice of freedom is a delusion. Idealism says the voice that tells of bondage is delusion. Vedanta says you are free and not free at the same time; never free on the earthly plane, but ever free on the spiritual.

Vivekananda

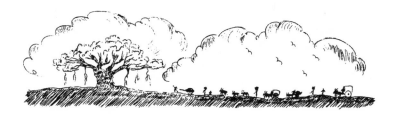

Who but the fool will choose his death rather than strive
with fate to bend it to his will?

S.Y.

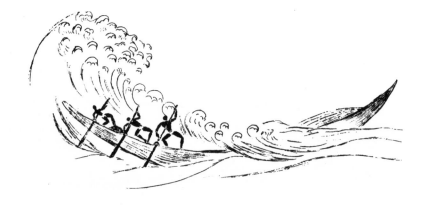

External cleansing means keeping the body clean; an unclean man will never become a Yogi. Inner cleansing, however, is also necessary. Inner cleanliness is naturally more valuable than outer cleanliness, but both are essential, for the latter without the former is to no avail.

Vivekananda

Hatha Yoga is not the ultimate goal. Hatha Yoga makes us aware that the body with its inestimable qualities is everything that we have in life; for we enter this world naked and leave it naked. For that reason we must get the best out of our body. The more we strive to unfold the perfections of the body, the more quickly our mental capacities unfold: power of concentration, memory, will-power and resolution. The blessing of Hatha Yoga is threefold: health, well-being and long life.

S.Y.

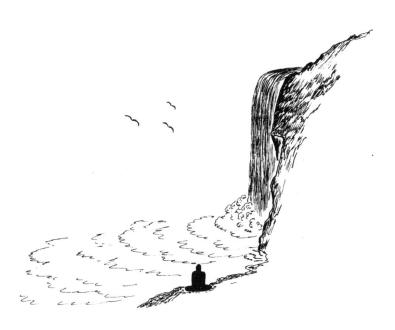

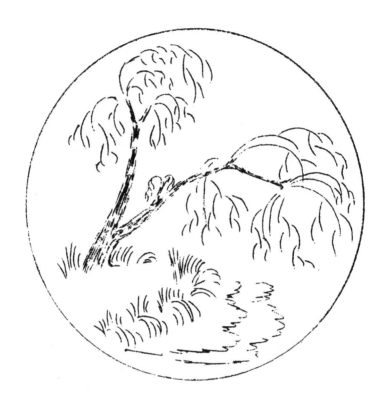

A Samnyasini (an itinerant mendicant nun dedicated to poverty) once came to the court of King Janaka. The King bowed before her, averting his eyes from her face. When the Samnyasini noticed this, she said: 'How strange, O Janaka, that you are still so afraid of woman! He who has attained complete knowledge (Jnana) becomes a childlike being—for him there is no longer any difference between the sexes.'

Ramakrishna

When Rama was enlightened by the teaching of his guru, he resolved to renounce the world. His father Dasaratha sent the sage Vasishtha to him to teach him. Vasishtha found Rama in a state of utter calm. 'Rama,' he said, 'let us first talk before you forsake the world. I ask you: is the world anything else but God? If so, you are free to renounce it.' Reflecting on these words the Prince realised that it was God whom he perceived as both manifested world and unmanifested Self, and that everything rests in His Being. Thus Rama fell silent.

Sri Ramakrishna

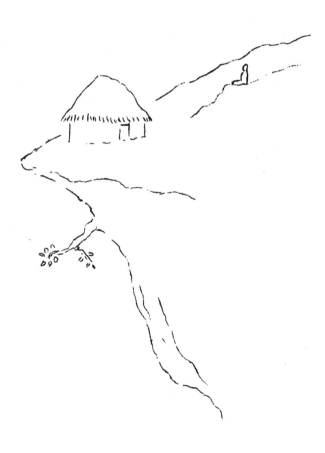

All that we are is the result of what we have thought: it is founded on our thoughts, it is made up of our thoughts. If a man speaks or acts with an evil thought, pain follows as the wheel follows the foot of the ox that draws the carriage.

All that we are is the result of what we have thought: it is founded on our thoughts, it is made up of our thoughts. If a man speaks or acts with a pure thought, happiness follows, like a shadow that never leaves him.

'He abused me, he beat me, he defeated me, he robbed me'—in those who harbour such thoughts hatred will never cease.

'He abused me, he beat me, he defeated me, he robbed me'—in those who do not harbour such thoughts hatred will cease.

For hatred does not cease by hatred at any time: hatred ceases by love—this is an old rule.

The world does not know that we must all come to an end here; but those who know it, their quarrels cease at once.

He who lives looking for pleasures only, his senses uncontrolled, immoderate in his food, idle and weak, Mara (the tempter) will certainly overthrow him, as the wind throws down a weak tree.

He who lives without looking for pleasures, his senses well controlled, moderate in his food, faithful and strong, him Mara will certainly not overthrow, any more than the wind throws down a rocky mountain.

They who imagine truth in untruth, and see untruth in truth, never arrive at truth, but follow vain desires.

They who know truth in truth, and untruth in untruth, arrive at truth, and follow true desires.

As rain breaks through an ill-thatched house, passion will break through an unreflecting mind.

As rain does not break through a well-thatched house, passion will not break through a well-reflecting mind.

The evil-doer mourns in this world, and he mourns in the next; he mourns in both. He mourns and suffers when he sees the evil result of his own work.

The virtuous man delights in this world, and he delights in the next; he delights in both. He delights and rejoices, when he sees the purity of his own work.

(The Dhammapada. The Teachings of Lord Buddha)

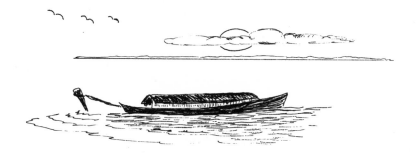

Prince Wen asked: 'Did you have a teacher?'
Dsi Fang said: 'Oh yes.'
'And who was your teacher?'
Dsi Fang said: 'Master Schun von Ostweiler.'
Prince Wen said: 'Why is it then that you have never quoted him?'
Dsi Fang said: 'He is a man who has attained the true being. By outward appearances a man, in reality, however, like heaven. He freely adapts to the world, yet disguises his true being. He is pure, yet lets all creatures do as they please. If they lack good SENSE, he is exemplary in his behaviour in order to rouse them. He causes men's selfish thoughts to disappear. But none of his words may be quoted.'

After Dsi Fang had departed, Prince Wen sat for a whole day in speechless torpidity. Then he called to one of his advisers in attendance and said to him: 'How infinitely superior to us is a man who possesses full LIFE! Until now I considered it the supreme achievement to utter the words of holy wisdom and to perform the works of love and duty. Now that I have heard of Dsi Fang's master, however, my body is limp and can no longer move, my lips are closed and can no longer speak. What I have learned is in reality no more than dust and earth. My country, alas, is in truth only a burden to me.'

Juang Dsi

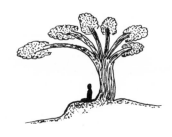

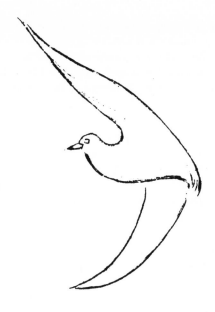

When you entered this world, Oh Tulsi, the world laughed with joy—but you wept. Now that you are in the world, live in such a way that when the time comes for you to leave this world, the world will weep—but you will depart in laughter.

Tulsidas

I went to the river to meet my thoughts alone,
And with the running waters
My thoughts, they too did run.
I watched their haste, the forms they took,
Their size, their shape, their hues.
And then I laughed
To see the river rob them one by one
And drown them in her watery bed.
When all my thoughts were gone
We were alone,
The river and I,
Just we two.

S.Y.

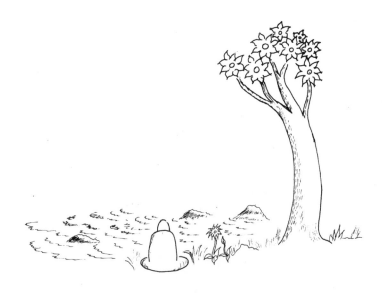

Boatman, take me to yonder shore,
'Tis there I live,
'Tis there I'll go,
To breathe once more
The air I breathed
Before I wandered to this shore.
'Tis Eternity's land,
A land without a shore,
Eternity I'll have,
And no more.

S.Y.

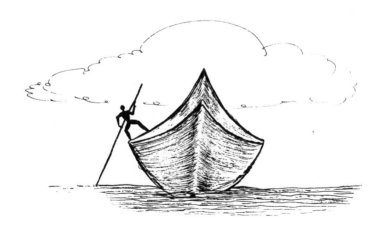

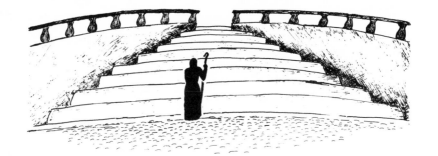

Ah, these weather-beaten steps of time where no footprints remain but only the memory of yesterday's pleasure turned into today's pain. Youth ascends the hoary steps of age and bids adieu to earthly shores, awakening at last from the dream-spell of creation called life and death.

S.Y.

The Beginning

'Where have I come from, where did you discover me?'
the baby asked its mother.

She answered half crying, half laughing, and clasping the
baby to her breast,

'You were hidden in my heart as its desire, my darling.

You were in the dolls of my childhood's games; and when
with clay

I made the image of my god every morning, I made and
unmade you then.

You were enshrined with our household deity, in his
worship I worshipped you.

In all my hopes and my loves, in my life, in the life of my
mother you have lived.

In the lap of the deathless Spirit who rules our home you
have been nursed for ages.

When in girlhood my heart was opening its petals, you
hovered as a fragrance about it.

Your tender softness bloomed in my youthful limbs, like a
glow in the sky before the sunrise.

Heaven's first darling, twin-born with the morning light,
you have floated down the stream of the world's life, and
at last you have stranded on my heart.

As I gaze on your face, mystery overwhelms me; you who
belong to all have become mine.

For fear of losing you I hold you tight to my breast. What
magic has snared the world's treasure in these slender arms
of mine?'

Rabindranath Tagore

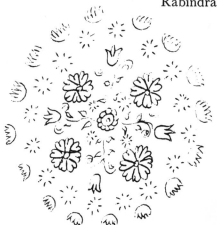

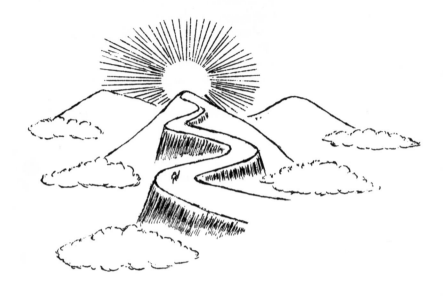

Alone I came into this world,
Alone I wander all my days.
My wanderings done yet still alone,
Homeward bound I pace my days
Toward the home that gave me birth.

S.Y.

LIST OF REFERENCES

The Complete Works of Swami Vivekananda, Advaita Ashrama, Mayavati Almora, Himalaya, India.

The Gospel of Sri Ramakrishna, Sri Ramakrishna Math, P.O. Belury Math, District Howrah, Bengal, India.

Talks with Sri Ramana Maharshi, T. N. Venkataraman, Sri Ramanasramam, Tiruvannamalai, S. India, India.

'Dhammapada' Translated by Dr Max Muller, quoted from *The Legacy of India*, G. T. Garrat, England.

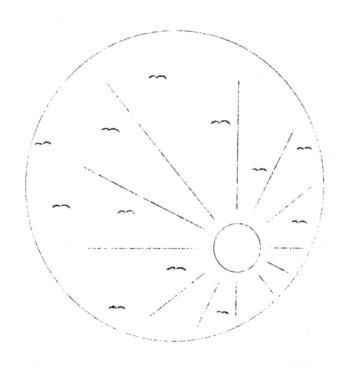